Spanaway Lake
High School

tourette syndrome

tourette syndrome

ELAINE LANDAU

Spanaway Lake
High School

A Venture Book
Franklin Watts
A Division of Grolier Publishing
New York London Hong Kong Sydney
Danbury, Connecticut

Interior Design by Molly Heron
Photographs ©: Ben Klaffke: 9, 10, 19, 25, 35, 36, 41, 43; Florida Marlins
Baseball: 47; Jag Entertainment: 56; North Wind Picture Archives: 58;

Library of Congress Cataloging-in-Publication Data

Landau, Elaine
    Tourette Syndrome / by Elaine Landau.
        p. cm. — (A Venture book)
    Includes bibliographical references and index.
    Summary: Describes causes, symptoms, and treatment
of Tourette Syndrome and explains the challenges faced
by people with the disorder.
    ISBN 0–531–11399–X
    1. Tourette Syndrome—Juvenile literature. [1. Tourette
Syndrome.] I. Title. II. Series.
RC375.L36 1998
616.8'3—dc21   97–48736
                                                   CIP
                                                    AC

contents

chapter 1

Tourette Syndrome

PEOPLE STARE AT YOU WHEREVER YOU GO. NO ONE SITS NEXT TO you on a bus or train. People often call you rude, offensive, and crazy, and there is nothing you can do to change their impression. This is what life can be like for someone with the inherited neurological disorder known as Tourette Syndrome (TS).

People with Tourette Syndrome are susceptible to repeated movements and vocalizations (sounds, words, or phrases) called tics. Tics are involuntary—they are unintentional and difficult or impossible to control. In mild cases, these tics may be infrequent and barely noticeable. In severe cases, the tics may be frequent and extremely disruptive. TS occurs worldwide, affecting people of all races and ethnic groups, although males are three to four times more likely than females to have the disorder.

To someone unfamiliar with Tourette Syndrome, the behavior of a person with the disorder might seem completely bizarre. The more common motor tics (bodily movements) include repeated winking or blinking, facial grimaces, sudden jerks of the head or shoulder, and similar unexpected movements of the hand and arm. People with Tourette Syndrome must contend with an array of vocal tics as well. A vocal tic may be a word or phrase, but it is just as likely to come out as throat clearing, sniffing, coughing, barking, clucking, hissing, or a popping sound.

SYMPTOMS OF TOURETTE SYNDROME

For someone to be diagnosed with Tourette Syndrome, the person must have exhibited a vocal tic and several motor tics over a period of time, although the two types of tics need not have occurred together. The diagnosis further requires that these symptoms have occurred at least several times a day (usually in bouts) and persisted for more than a year. The tics must also change in intensity over time and have appeared before the individual was eighteen years old.

The various tics associated with Tourette Syndrome are classified as either simple or complex. The National Institute of Neurological Disorders and Stroke describes simple motor tics as sudden brief movements that involve a limited number of muscle groups and are repetitive. Eye blinking, shoulder shrugging, head jerking, facial grimacing, sniffing, and twitching are examples of simple motor tics. Simple vocal tics are brief, meaningless sounds. Throat clearing or yelping are examples of simple vocal tics. Complex motor tics are movements involving several muscle groups. Pinching, punching, jumping, smelling objects, and repeatedly touching people or things are complex motor tics. Complex vocal tics are sounds, such as words or phrases, that appear to have meaning.

A person's tics rarely remain constant; they can change at any time for no apparent reason. The tics also vary in intensity. Most people with TS experience only mild symptoms, but a minority have severe tics that may interfere with going to school, keeping a job, or participating in social activities.

The most sensationalized type of vocal tic is coprolalia. People with this rare vocal tic involuntarily repeat obscenities or make other socially inappropriate com-

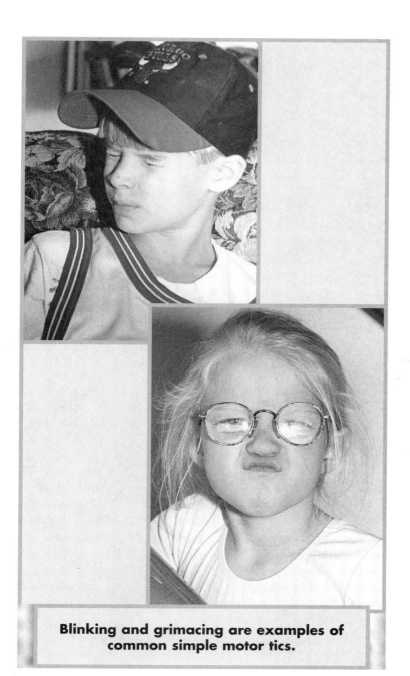

Blinking and grimacing are examples of common simple motor tics.

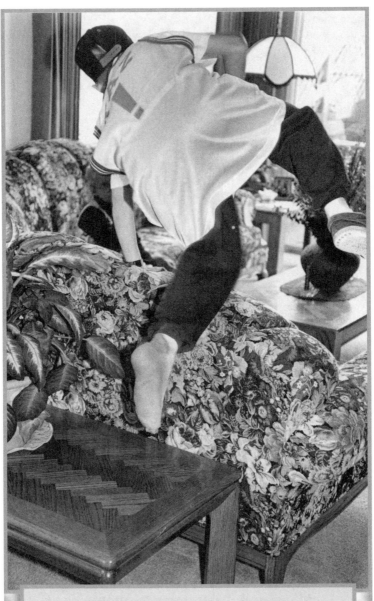

Jumping is a complex motor tic.

ments. Some people automatically associate this tic with Tourette Syndrome, but in reality, less than 15 percent of people with TS suffer from coprolalia.

Other complex vocal tics are palilalia and echolalia. With palilalia, a person repeats the last word or sound he or she has made. For example, the individual might say something like, "I'm going to my room, room, room." A person with echolalia repeats someone else's last word or phrase. If a teacher says "Please take your seat" to a student with this type of tic, the young person might repeat, "your seat, your seat, your seat."

Often, Tourette Syndrome first appears when a child is between seven and nine years old and intensifies during early adolescence (between twelve and fifteen years of age). Fortunately, the tics usually begin to diminish between the ages of sixteen and eighteen and continue to lessen in severity with age.

While the tics associated with the disorder are usually described as involuntary, many people with TS can temporarily suppress their tics. In most cases, the suppressed tics must be released at a later time, and these outbursts can be more severe than they would have been had they not been delayed. As one neurologist who has done extensive research on Tourette Syndrome explains, "Patients don't say, 'Gee, I don't know where that movement came from.' They are aware of their tics before they happen. They can suppress the urges, but the longer they do so, the more they feel the need for a massive catharsis."[1] Many people with TS compare the urge to release their tics to the irresistible need to sneeze or scratch a mosquito bite. One young man with Tourette Syndrome adds, "It's a feeling of having an itch on one's back you can't reach, that tension building. Then there's the symptom and the feeling of, 'Whew, it's out.'"[2]

Tics are the only symptoms that are part of the core definition of Tourette Syndrome, but other disorders frequently accompany TS. These include depression, anxiety, obsessive compulsive disorder (OCD), attention deficit hyperactivity disorder (ADHD), self-injurious behavior (such as lip biting, cheek biting, or banging one's head against hard objects), and aggression. These disorders appear much more often in people with TS than they do in the rest of the population. In many cases, the associated disorders are more difficult to live with than the tics.

PREVALENCE OF TOURETTE SYNDROME

At one time Tourette Syndrome was believed to be extremely rare, but this perception is changing. The National Institutes of Health estimates that about 100,000 people in the United States have full-blown TS. Other estimates show that one out of every thousand young American boys may have TS, while at least three times as many people display some TS symptoms.[3] Many health care experts think that the actual number may be even higher since numerous people with Tourette Syndrome are never correctly diagnosed, and many people with mild cases never need medical attention.

Dr. Ann Young, a neurologist at Harvard University and the chairperson of the Tourette Syndrome Association's Scientific Advisory Board, has further suggested that tics may be considerably more common than most people believe. She explains:

> If you go to any elementary school, up to a quarter of the children will have tics. . . . They roll their eyes, snap their fingers, smack their lips. But the tics tend to last just a few months, which implies that their brain circuits controlling movements are maturing. . . . In Tourette's patients, tics tend to come and go throughout life and to worsen with stress. But the same may be true of all of us. I watch people and see a lot of tics. It might be a little shoulder twitch, clearing the throat, tapping the fingers.

Whenever I give a lecture on Tourette's and mention this, I see people in the audience beginning to squirm. I think we can all relate to such experiences.[4]

LIVING WITH TOURETTE SYNDROME

While some people with TS can hold back their tics in public places, not everyone with Tourette Syndrome has this degree of control. And the act of suppressing tics can have unwanted side effects. The mother of a boy with Tourette Syndrome described the repercussions of trying to stop her son's tics as follows:

> I kept reminding him . . . "Tommy, don't do that. Stop it. You know, you're doing it again." And we actually got him to stop for a period of a day. And what I discovered was that at night when I went to check on him, he was ticcing in his sleep. He was just going absolutely wild. . . . He had held it in and it just had to come out. You cannot hold it back—it has to come out somehow, somewhere, and that's what it did. It came out in his sleep.[5]

People with Tourette Syndrome often find that not everyone will understand and be sympathetic to their condition. This is especially true in cases in which the individual with TS habitually insults, slanders, or uses profanity. Some have even been assaulted by people they unintentionally offended.

For a minority of individuals with very severe cases of TS, just getting through the day can be challenging. That is what it's like for Steve, a young man from Brookline, Massachusetts, whose tics interfere with most aspects of his daily life. At times he's been seen in department stores muttering bizarre remarks to no one in particular. Often he will make fun of people's names or utter profanities. Sometimes Steve involuntarily uses racial slurs, and he finds this tic particularly ironic considering the discrimination he has personally endured because of his disorder. "Living with Tourette's and the hell I've been through," says Steve, "the last thing in the world I would do is turn to discriminate against another individual."[6]

Many people who see Steve think he is insane or intoxicated and quickly distance themselves from him. And for Steve, the resulting isolation has been extremely demoralizing. As a child, before he was diagnosed with TS, Steve even had to cope with his own family's intolerance of his disorder. After telling him over and over to stop making an annoying sound, his parents did not understand their son's reply of, "I can't help it." Steve recalls, "I'd get dragged into another room and beaten with a broomstick for a while."[7]

As an adult, Steve's TS symptoms have prevented him from finding work. In recent years he's applied for at least seventy-five positions and been turned down every time. For a while he lived off a small inheritance, spending much of his time on the street. When the money ran out, he was forced to go on public assistance.

Steve's life has been unusually difficult because he has a very severe case of Tourette Syndrome. Most others with the disorder have milder symptoms. Also, Steve's condition has worsened as he has aged. For the majority of those with Tourette Syndrome, the opposite is true. Most individuals with Tourette Syndrome hold down jobs, have families, and function well within their communities. Nevertheless, at one time or another, many people with Tourette Syndrome have experienced some type of discrimination as the result of their often misunderstood disorder.

chapter 2

A Neurological Disorder

THE FIRST DOCUMENTED CASE OF TOURETTE SYNDROME WAS observed by the 19th-century French neurologist Jean-Marc Itard. His patient was a French noblewoman, the Marquise de Dampierre, who began exhibiting motor tics when she was seven years old. Shortly thereafter, the girl developed vocal tics including screams and high-pitched cries. By the time she was nine, the child would shout out profanities accompanied by obscene gestures. Sadly, the girl's broad range of behavior problems prompted her family to force her into isolation. She spent the rest of her life in seclusion. Her involuntary outbursts of cursing and screaming continued until her death at the age of eighty-five.

More than a half century after Dr. Itard's death, another French physician, Georges Gilles de la Tourette, produced detailed case histories of several patients with remarkably similar symptoms to those of the Marquise de Dampierre. Tourette had even traced the course of the Marquise's illness in her later years of life. Having definitively identified the syndrome and its various symptoms, his name was given to the disorder.

At the time, little was known about the causes of the syndrome or how to treat those affected. People with the disorder were believed to be mentally ill. Unfortunately, the precise cause of Tourette Syndrome remains mysterious, but researchers now know that it is an inherited physical disorder caused by an abnormality of certain genes. This abnormality disrupts the way the brain processes chemicals called neurotransmitters, which carry signals between nerve cells. The main neurotransmitters believed to be affected are called serotonin, norepinephrine, and dopamine.

DOPAMINE AND TOURETTE SYNDROME

Some research suggests that tics may be caused by an oversensitivity to normal amounts of dopamine produced in the brain. Patients who are extremely sensitive to this chemical appear to have the most severe tics— various parts of their bodies twitch throughout the day, and they continually voice meaningless phrases. People with Tourette Syndrome whose sensitivity to dopamine is closer to normal tend to have milder tics, such as occasional blinking or shrugging.

These research results grew out of a study at the National Institute of Mental Health in which five sets of identical twins with Tourette Syndrome were examined. In each case, one twin's symptoms were significantly more severe than the other's, even though they had identical genes. The researchers examined the behavior of the twins and used sophisticated technology to generate images of their brains. These images showed differences in a part of the brain called the caudate nucleus.

The caudate nucleus acts as a brake to curb certain motor impulses. The effect of the caudate nucleus is regulated by dopamine. When dopamine binds to the caudate nucleus, it diminishes the ability of the caudate nucleus to control motor impulses. When the brain is acting normally, just enough dopamine binds to the caudate nucleus to ensure that motor impulses remain at the optimum level. If too much dopamine binds, however, the caudate nucleus cannot control motor impulses effectively, and a person becomes susceptible to tics.

The images of the twins' brains showed that in each case, more dopamine binds to the caudate nucleus of the twin with the more severe tics. But what makes one twin more sensitive to dopamine than the other? Dr. Daniel Weinberger, one of the scientists who conducted the study, admits that, at present, medical science cannot account for the difference in the caudate nucleuses of the identical twins. However, doctors suspect that it may be connected to the children's prenatal (prior to birth) experience. When both twins have Tourette Syndrome, the one with the lower birth weight generally has more severe tics. It is further suspected that the intensity of the tics may also result from stress. Weinberger noted that "while twins have the same genes they are not the same person."[1] Often, one twin proves to be more susceptible to the tensions and stresses of everyday life.

INHERITING TOURETTE SYNDROME

Researchers know that Tourette Syndrome is a genetic disorder passed down through families. TS can be transmitted to a son or daughter by a parent of either sex. A person with a family history of Tourette Syndrome, however, doesn't necessarily inherit the disorder. Children of parents with Tourette Syndrome have about a 50 percent chance of inheriting the gene (or genes) that causes the disorder.* Even among those who do inherit the gene (or genes), some will develop TS, some will show no signs of TS, and some will display other tic disorders that are not severe enough to be classified as Tourette Syndrome. Overall, only about 10 percent of those who inherit the gene (or genes) will have symptoms severe enough to require medical attention. Some

---

* It is not yet known whether Tourette Syndrome is caused by a single gene or a combination of genes.

people with Tourette Syndrome show no family history of the disorder. The cause of these cases, known as sporadic Tourette Syndrome, is unknown.

Children who inherit Tourette Syndrome from their mother or father do not necessarily display the same symptoms with the same intensity as their parent. The duration, number, and types of tics vary significantly. A parent with severe symptoms can have a child who has mild tics, or the reverse may be true.

If a child inherits the gene (or genes) that causes Tourette Syndrome, the chances of showing signs of a tic disorder depend tremendously on the sex of the child. Though not all boys with the gene (or genes) will develop full-blown TS, almost all (99 percent) will show some susceptibility to tics during their lives. By contrast, only 56 to 70 percent of girls with the gene (or genes) will be susceptible to tics.

CO-OCCURRING DISORDERS

As noted earlier, several disorders are known to be more common in people with Tourette Syndrome than in the rest of the population. The high incidence of these disorders in people with TS leads scientists to believe that they have related causes. The disorders that frequently accompany Tourette Syndrome include those discussed below. Some people with Tourette Syndrome have two or three of these disorders.

Obsessive Compulsive Disorder

It is estimated that more than 50 percent of those with TS also exhibit obsessive compulsive disorder (OCD) symptoms. According to the National Institute of Mental Health, "The individual who suffers from obsessive compulsive behavior becomes trapped in a pattern of repetitive thoughts and behaviors that are senseless and distressing but extremely difficult to overcome."[2] These

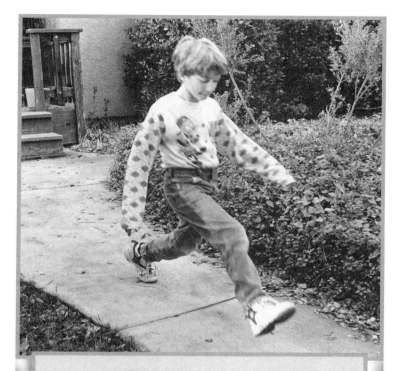

Most people, at some point in their lives, perform compulsive behaviors. Simple behaviors such as avoiding the cracks on a pathway may be compulsive. Only when obsessive or compulsive behaviors become excessive and intrusive are they considered to be a disorder.

individuals claim that unwanted ideas or impulses repeatedly well up in their minds. Among the most common of these unpleasant thought patterns are persistent fears that harm may come to a loved one or themselves, an unreasonable belief that they have a terrible illness, or a relentless need to do things perfectly.

19

People with OCD also often feel compelled to perform certain acts in a precise, ritualistic manner. This may include repeatedly washing their hands, checking to see if the door is locked, insisting on wearing a specific hat in a certain way, or having only brown shoes in their closet. Young people with obsessive compulsive disorder may need to sit in the same seat every time they go to the movies or perhaps endlessly recheck their homework for possible errors. These repetitive behaviors are generally intended to ward off some imagined harm to themselves or others. Although performing these behaviors may somewhat diminish the person's anxiety, the relief is only temporary.

Obsessive compulsive disorder can hinder a child's functioning both at school and in social settings. Continually repeating specific behaviors can be time consuming and distracting. A young person who must return to his or her room over and over again to make certain that nothing has been left behind may be late for school most days. Similarly, a child who feels compelled to repeatedly count the pencils on his teacher's desk during a test period may not be able to complete the exam in the allotted time.

One mother remembers what life was like for her young daughter who had both OCD and TS:

> When she was seven, Joan's tics were causing her lots of problems. She had this cough—she did it fifty or a hundred times a day. She would also squint her eyes and jerk her shoulder. This was enough of a problem, but on top of that she had this hand-washing routine. I couldn't count how many times a day she washed her hands. She had to have a clean towel each time and she was wild over germs. She thought everything had germs; we had to cover our plates before each meal, and if someone coughed or sneezed in the kitchen or at the table, she wouldn't eat.[3]

Attention Deficit Hyperactivity Disorder

Another disorder that commonly occurs with Tourette Syndrome is attention deficit hyperactivity disorder (ADHD). Individuals with this problem tend to be easily distracted and have difficulty concentrating for any length of time. Some young people with ADHD may constantly fidget and squirm in their seats at school, while others may not be able to remain seated quietly for more than a few minutes at a time. Other symptoms of ADHD include interrupting others, talking continuously, finding it difficult to wait in line, frequently misplacing things, having difficulty following directions, and seeming not to listen when spoken to. Youths with this disorder often find it hard to complete assignments or chores and frequently switch from one unfinished task to another. Attention deficit disorder (ADD) is a similar disorder that also frequently occurs with TS. Individuals with ADD display all the symptoms described here excluding the high activity level.

In children with TS who have ADHD (or ADD), the ADHD symptoms usually appear prior to the Tourette Syndrome tics. Some medications frequently prescribed for ADHD can worsen tics in patients with TS, so prescriptions must be checked and changed in some situations.

Learning Disabilities

Having Tourette Syndrome does not affect a person's intelligence in any way. Yet even an extremely gifted child with Tourette Syndrome can have some form of learning problems. Approximately one-third of those with TS have a learning disability. Such students may experience difficulties with reading, writing, or math. At times, TS tics such as head jerking or eye blinking can make reading difficult and thus hinder learning in other subjects.

Sleep Disorders

It is not uncommon for people with Tourette Syndrome to experience sleep disorders. These may include having difficulty falling asleep, being unable to sleep through the night, talking in one's sleep, and even sleepwalking.

Problems with Impulse Control

About one-fourth of the children who have Tourette Syndrome also have a "short fuse" when it comes to anger and impulsive behavior. These children may get into fights or destroy other people's property with little provocation. At times they may turn their rage inward and engage in self-destructive behavior. Following such outbursts, they are often embarrassed by their actions and sorry about what they did. Yet they continue to find it difficult to control their impulses. Research shows that aggressive behavior is most common in youths with TS who also have ADHD. In some cases, aggressive behavior intensifies as tics worsen, but this isn't true for everyone.

Doctors still can't completely explain the relationship between aggressive behavior and TS. It may have a biological basis or may be at least partly due to the increased stress of having to deal with the academic and social pressures resulting from a severe case of Tourette Syndrome.

DIAGNOSIS

Diagnosing Tourette Syndrome can sometimes be tricky. At this time there is still no specific blood or neurological test that can definitively determine whether or not someone has Tourette Syndrome. Instead, the diagnosis is usually arrived at through an observation of the patient's symptoms and an evaluation of the person's family history. Some physicians also have their patients undergo a full battery of tests, including magnetic resonance imaging (MRI), computerized tomography (CT), electroencephalogram (EEG) scans, and certain blood tests. These tests are given to rule out other possible causes for the symptoms.

Studies reveal that an accurate diagnosis of Tourette Syndrome is too often delayed because many doctors are unfamiliar with the condition. Also, TS symptoms can easily be misinterpreted, causing children with Tourette Syndrome to be misunderstood at home, in school, and even at their physician's office. Because TS symptoms frequently wax and wane (increase and decrease) in severity—and can sometimes be repressed for at least short periods—a young person may never exhibit tics in his or her doctor's presence. Hopefully, diagnosis will improve as more precise diagnostic tools are developed and awareness of the disorder increases.

TREATMENT

While there is presently no cure for Tourette Syndrome, some forms of treatment are frequently helpful. The type of treatment usually depends on the severity of the disorder. The majority of people with Tourette Syndrome have mild symptoms and generally do not need medication. However, because stress can worsen tics, these individuals often find it helpful to learn stress reduction techniques. And whether their symptoms are mild or severe, people with TS also find that individual counseling can help them cope with the disorder and feel better about themselves. As one parent of a boy with TS describes:

> Kids with TS need counseling as they approach adolescence. An eleven- or twelve-year-old wants to be just like his peers, and having TS sets him apart. Lots of anger and frustration builds up. They ask questions like, "Will girls ever like me?" "Will I be able to get a job when I get older?" Counseling

gives them an outlet to express all of their feelings and it helps to build up self-esteem and eventual acceptance of themselves.[4]

In cases in which a person's TS symptoms impair his or her daily functioning, a number of medications can help alleviate tics. No single drug works for everyone, however, and controlling very severe TS symptoms can be complicated. Unfortunately, even the most effective medications cannot reduce every patient's tics. In addition, many of these drugs can have unpleasant side effects.

The medications most frequently used by TS patients to control motor and vocal tics are known as neuroleptic drugs. They work by blocking the neurotransmitter dopamine, which people with Tourette Syndrome are highly sensitive to. When treating TS, the most commonly used neuroleptic drugs are Haldol (haloperidol) and Orap (pimozide). While Haldol and Orap reduce tics, both medications produce negative side effects that worsen if the drug dosage is increased. The various side effects can include restlessness, muscular rigidity, slowed movement, and a lack of facial expression. In rare cases, patients who take neuroleptics for an extended period of time may develop an involuntary movement disorder known as tardive dyskinesia. Often, these movements involve the patient's tongue and mouth muscles. Usually, this disorder will disappear once the medication is discontinued.

Catapres (clonidine) is sometimes used instead of neuroleptic drugs to treat tics. A number of studies indicate that this drug is more effective in eliminating motor tics than vocal tics. Common side effects that can occur with Catapres include fatigue, dry mouth, irritability, dizziness, headaches, and insomnia.

When medicating a patient, a doctor will try to prescribe the drug that will provide the most benefits for the particular individual with the least side effects. Usually

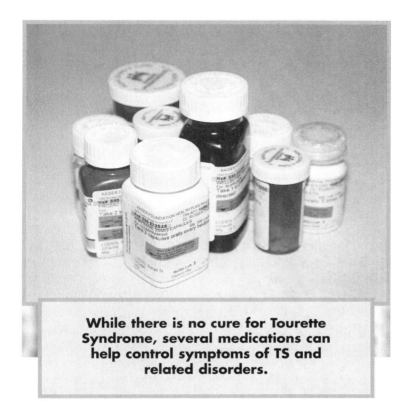

While there is no cure for Tourette Syndrome, several medications can help control symptoms of TS and related disorders.

the patient starts with a low dosage that can be gradually increased if necessary.

In many cases, the disorders that may accompany Tourette Syndrome are never severe enough to require treatment. Sometimes, however, these disorders can disrupt a person's life more than the tics. Fortunately, many of these other disorders can also be treated when necessary.

Medications for attention deficit hyperactivity disorder (ADHD) curb restlessness and enhance the individual's attention span. Yet, as with the medications to reduce tics, the effectiveness of these drugs varies greatly from patient to patient, and they may produce unacceptable side effects. Stimulants such as Ritalin (methylphenidate) are commonly used to treat attention deficit hyperactivity disorder. Unfortunately, this type of drug has been known to worsen tics in people with Tourette Syndrome. If this occurs, the drug will usually be discontinued and other medications substituted.

In such cases, medications known as tricyclic antidepressants may be tried. Among these, Norpramin (desipramine) and Anafranil (clomipramine) are the most commonly prescribed for people with Tourette Syndrome. These may be taken in conjunction with medications to reduce tics. Anafranil and another tricyclic antidepressant known as Prozac (fluoxetine) are also sometimes helpful in reducing obsessive compulsive disorder traits.

It is extremely important that individuals taking these drugs be monitored by a physician. At times, the medication may need to be increased, decreased, or changed to counteract side effects. Patients should not abruptly stop taking these medications unless directed to do so by a physician. Doctors generally prefer to gradually withdraw a drug.

The medications described here are just a few of the drugs used to treat Tourette Syndrome and some of the related disorders. Doctors often try new drugs for treating TS as they are developed. When properly used, the right medication can make a tremendous difference for some individuals who have found other treatments ineffective.

RESEARCH

Researchers are continuing to examine the ways in which dopamine and other neurotransmitters contribute to the symptoms of Tourette Syndrome. At this time, research on Tourette Syndrome is also being conducted in the the following areas.

Genetic Studies

In each cell of your body, you have 50,000 to 100,000 genes. These genes contain information about your physical appearance and all other inherited traits. Inherited diseases and disorders, such as Tourette Syndrome, are also passed down through genes.

Genes are made up of a substance called deoxyribonucleic acid, or DNA. The makeup of your DNA is almost exactly the same as the DNA of every other human being. If you could compare all your DNA to the DNA of a classmate, you would find only very small differences. In general, these differences are normal, and they account for the physical differences in people. Some differences are not normal, however, and may be the source of a genetic disorder such as Tourette Syndrome.

Scientists hope to isolate the particular gene (or genes) that causes Tourette Syndrome by detecting a specific DNA abnormality common to all people with the disorder. Unfortunately, this is an extremely difficult and painstaking process. DNA is so small, and there is so much of it in the human body, that isolating a particular abnormality can take many years. Nevertheless, the search for the gene (or genes) that causes TS is underway.

Researchers are conducting studies involving large families in which members spanning several generations have Tourette Syndrome. They hope to find a DNA abnormality that all family members with TS share. Researchers could then pinpoint the specific gene (or genes) that causes Tourette Syndrome.

Genetic research is an important part of the attempt to learn more about Tourette Syndrome. Locating the gene (or genes) for TS would be extremely helpful in improving techniques for identifying who is at risk for inheriting the disorder. In addition, it may help researchers better understand how the disorder develops, improve present diagnostic techniques, and devise more effective treatments.

Environmental Studies

Research projects are underway to learn more about the role the environment plays in Tourette Syndrome. For example, how important is a person's environment in determining whether someone at high risk for Tourette Syndrome actually develops the disorder? Also, do environmental factors, such as stress or taking certain medications, influence the severity of TS symptoms? The answers to these questions and others may help people with TS modify their environment to alleviate some of their symptoms.

chapter 3

Coping with
Tourette Syndrome

WHEN I WAS NINE YEARS OLD, AN IMP TOOK UP RESIDENCE
in me. One afternoon he prodded the left side of
my face from the inside, causing my lips to purse
and curl askew toward my squinting left eye.
Within a few days he was making mischief
throughout my being. Without yet knowing why, I
rapidly blinked and shrugged. I grunted. I threw
back my head and squeaked while my fists
snatched my bruised abdomen.[1]   —Mark

Although he didn't know it at the time, Mark had
Tourette Syndrome. Sadly, he had to contend with
more than just vocal and motor tics. He had to fight
self-destructive urges to jump from a second-story win-
dow or thrust his fingers into the blades of an electric
cake mixer.

Although Mark had a severe case of TS as a child, it
went undiagnosed. For many years he dealt with the em-
barrassment and shame resulting from his symptoms
without knowing why he acted as he did. When his
mother took him to the doctor, the physician made light of
the boy's tics, simply saying, "He's a nervous child. They're
just bad habits."[2] Then, when Mark was thirty-five, he visited a doctor to complain about a joint pain that had developed as a result of twenty-six years of ticcing. The doc-

tor recognized the symptoms of Tourette Syndrome, and Mark was finally diagnosed with the disorder.

Even today, too many young children with Tourette Syndrome are not properly diagnosed. Prior to an accurate diagnosis of Tourette Syndrome, a child may feel alone and unable to control many important aspects of his or her life. "Children mocked me and my father often informed me of a tic by angrily slapping my head," remembers a young man with Tourette Syndrome. "Shunned by other children and occasionally my own father, I felt like an outsider. I was ashamed and lonely and full of self-pity. I believed I was already living in hell."[3]

At times, some people's symptoms have even jeopardized their safety. One thirteen-year-old boy with Tourette Syndrome remembers involuntarily shouting racial slurs in a rest room. "We were at a [Houston] Rockets game because that's my favorite team," the young teen recalls. "And I was in the rest room. And a kid came in and I . . . I yelled a cuss word. . . . I said [a] racial slur. And he punched me in the stomach, and my mom found me leaning up against a wall."[4]

Having a child with Tourette Syndrome can be extremely difficult for parents and other family members. The mother of the boy who was punched in the lavatory was determined never to let it happen again. When her son had to use a public rest room, she asked an adult male to accompany him. Though it was sometimes awkward, she believed it was essential to have someone there to defuse potentially volatile situations.

Parents who aren't aware of the neurological basis for their child's actions sometimes believe their child is just misbehaving. To make matters worse, no amount of pleading or punishment seems to have a positive effect. In some cases it takes years before children are properly diagnosed, and during that time these young people may be wrongfully labeled and ridiculed by those around them. Some students have even been unfairly expelled from school and harshly disciplined for symptoms beyond their control.

One parent explains how their incomplete knowledge of TS proved emotionally costly for her son:

> We knew about TS, the lip smacking and the way he flipped his head like he was trying to get the hair out of his eyes, but we didn't know about the echoing. He started repeating the last two or three words of each sentence. At first it was a whisper and then out loud. We had four very tough months before someone told us that the repeating (by this time he would repeat things we said out loud) was also a part of TS. He got into so much trouble at school because of this, and we weren't able to help him at home because we didn't know.[5]

Desperate parents have even tried to have their children exorcised (rid of evil spirits) by the church. Incredibly, one young boy with TS who had no idea what was happening to him was relieved to hear his Sunday school teacher suggest that he was possessed by the devil. At least that was an explanation for his outlandish behavior. He remembers the incident this way:

> [My Sunday school teacher] said while glaring at me, "He [Jesus] following his stay in the wilderness . . . cured the lunatics and people with palsy and cast demons out of the possessed.". . . Her implication made sense to me. And despite my hatred of whatever made me tic, I was rather relieved to hear it was a demon. . . . After all, didn't that mean that my tics were caused by a sort of supernatural tapeworm and not by my own weakness?[6]

In another case, a young girl continually prayed to God to cure her of TS. While religious faith can prove helpful for some in coping with TS, this small child felt that God had abandoned her when her prayers didn't reduce her symptoms. One day, her parents found her in their bedroom crying and praying, "Please, God, take away my Tourette's. Take away my cussing. I've asked you and asked you, and you must not love me because you don't take them away."[7]

Those unfamiliar with TS often need time to become accustomed to the disorder's more disconcerting symptoms. This is evident in the experience of one mother who grew tired of missing parties and other family gatherings because of her son Phillip's TS symptoms. This woman and her husband decided to bring Phillip to her office party. To help her coworkers know what to expect beforehand, the woman allowed them to listen to a telephone call from her son over the company's speakerphone. As always, Phillip cursed a number of times during the conversation. However, the woman had wanted her coworkers to hear him so that no one would be shocked or offended if he spoke similarly at the party. After the boy hung up she told her fellow employees, "This is my son. He has Tourette's. We're going to have this at the party, and I want you to understand how he's going to behave." She recalls, "Everyone laughed and thought it was cool. But when we got to the party Phillip called the director a slut. And even though they [her coworkers] knew that [he had TS] and had been forewarned, they just could not believe that he was behaving this way."[8]

At this point, the woman found herself in an awkward situation. She and her husband were not sure whether it would be best for them to stay or leave the party. She didn't feel she should apologize for her son's behavior because she had explained its neurological cause ahead of time. But she was disappointed in her coworkers, who stared at her son with their mouths open in disbelief. She sums up her experience with people who do not understand TS this way:

> I always say he has Tourette's. If [I] walk up to . . .
> you in public and say, "My son has Tourette

Syndrome and he curses and doesn't want to" . . . you'll say, "OK!" And then I'll say, "Do you know what Tourette's is?" And I'll bet you a hundred-dollar bill that most [people] . . . have no idea what I'm talking about. But they won't admit that they don't know either.[9]

COPING AS A FAMILY

Coworkers and acquaintances aren't the only ones who react unfavorably to the difficulties of Tourette Syndrome. Some parents have found it exceedingly hard to cope with their child's disorder, and in extreme cases some have experienced despair. Although most people with TS lead full and productive lives, at first the situation may seem hopeless and unbearable. One mother who felt this way reports that she momentarily considered resorting to desperate measures:

> When they told me [that my son] had Tourette Syndrome . . . I went home and I felt really depressed about it. . . . And I [thought] . . . maybe I ought to take him out and take me too. But then I realized that God has us here for a purpose . . . to teach other people that you can live. We're not going to die from having Tourette's. . . . We've got things that we can do . . . things we can do for our society to educate them. And so, for some reason, we are here.[10]

Although contemplating suicide is a very rare reaction, it's not unusual for the parents and siblings of someone with Tourette Syndrome, as well as the affected individual, to experience a broad range of emotions while coming to terms with the disorder. Often reactions will vary depending on the severity of the symptoms. Those with extremely mild cases of TS may have to make few adjustments. Usually they are able to maintain friendships, attend regular school classes, and participate fully in various sporting and social activities.

However, for youths with severe tics, the situation may be quite different. These children and their families may have to accept that their lives will change considerably. At first, the child and parents may try to deny the diagnosis, hoping that somehow there is another explanation for the behavior. It may be especially hard for a child who has been teased or rejected by classmates to hear that there is no cure for Tourette Syndrome and that the symptoms will probably get worse before they get better.

After finding that Tourette Syndrome is usually hereditary, parents may feel guilty for having passed TS on to their offspring. If no one remembers anyone having TS symptoms in their families, they may spend hours questioning older family members about relatives who might have been thought of as eccentric. At times, other family members may become extremely defensive. As a parent of a young girl with TS notes, "When I told my parents about our daughter's TS, they said, 'It couldn't have come from our side of the family, by God!'" Even after learning the facts about TS, another child's grandmother was still unable to accept that the problem was hereditary. She was overheard saying, "I still wonder if he could have caught it from the dog."[11]

FINDING SUPPORT

Instead of looking for someone to blame, it's far more beneficial for families to focus on the future. It's often helpful for the family to become involved in a local support group for people with Tourette Syndrome and their families. At these gatherings, youths with TS can meet other young people with the disorder who lead happy, fulfilling lives. Families will also be able to attend various functions and holiday gatherings with people who understand the disorder. It's often a relief for families to

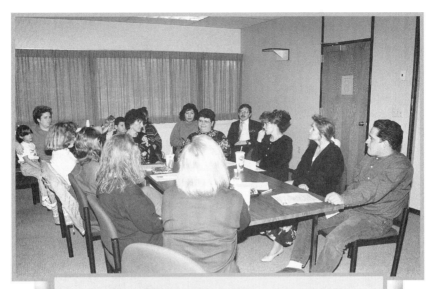

A support group for people with Tourette Syndrome and their families is often an invaluable resource for coping with the disorder.

find that whatever they are feeling has probably been felt by many others before them. They are also likely to get valuable advice from people who have already overcome the most common obstacles.

Unfortunately, TS symptoms often tend to be worst during adolescence—precisely the time when young people desperately long to be just like their peers and not stand out in any negative way. Therefore, it's especially important that their families and close friends learn as much as they can about TS to provide a firm support base for these young people. Many youths feel forced to suppress their tics when they are away from home to avoid the stares and ridicule of others. So it's essential they be allowed to relax at home—releasing their tics with no

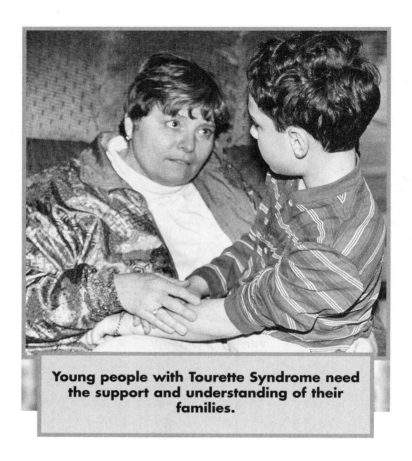

Young people with Tourette Syndrome need the support and understanding of their families.

fear of being blamed or criticized. Knowing that the people closest to them love and accept them regardless of their symptoms can provide a much-needed boost to their feelings about themselves. One mother describes her efforts to show her son that she would always be there for him:

> Once when he was thrashing around on the kitchen floor, I held him—so he thrashed me around with him! But I told him I was there and

wouldn't leave him, and that I loved him and he was a good little boy. That was what he needed then, and I had to stay with him for nearly an hour. It made me more determined than ever not to ever let him down, but to support and reassure him and be there.[12]

Young people with Tourette Syndrome often have low self-esteem after hearing for years that they are "weird," "nasty," or "crazy." Until they gain a healthy sense of self-respect, it is frequently difficult for them to win the acceptance and friendship of those around them.

SCHOOL AND TOURETTE SYNDROME

Parents can help their child feel comfortable in school by ensuring that their child's school counselors and teachers are aware of the neurological basis of TS and have devised a suitable plan for the student's education. No single approach to learning will work for every young person with TS. A team of qualified professionals must assess the student's capabilities and determine how that young person can best achieve his or her potential.

For example, while some students may do best in special schools, even those with moderate or severe TS symptoms can function quite well in a regular classroom. Sometimes, minor adjustments may be necessary. A teacher may need to learn to ignore a student's tics because calling attention to them may generate stress, which tends to make tics worse. The other students in the class will likely follow their teacher's example and be more tolerant of a classmate with TS.

At times, teachers may seat a student with TS where he or she can quickly exit the room to release tics. Being given a degree of privacy in dealing with the tics offers the young person some sense of control. And students who do not have to spend all their energy trying to hold back TS tics are free to concentrate on their class work.

It is also a good idea to educate the child's classmates about what TS actually is. This may mean having a parent or health-care professional visit the classroom to speak about what it's like to have TS. It is crucial for people to realize that when someone has coprolalia the loud noises or inappropriate remarks he or she may make are not done deliberately. "When this symptom is explained," a therapist notes, "it is most important to stress the involuntary and meaningless nature of the words spoken. . . . It is essential to explain that the outbursts are not directed toward any one person, as some people incorrectly assume. Handing out literature that discusses coprolalia helps to give your explanation credibility."[13] Some teachers have made learning about TS a class assignment. Hopefully this knowledge will lead to a more understanding and tolerant school environment.

After learning about Tourette Syndrome, some students may act more sympathetically, but this will not always be the case. Those with TS will probably have to learn to ignore teasing or ridicule from insensitive peers and seek out true friends. This is often easier said than done, since the taunting is likely to become worse before fading out. However, when bullies realize their taunts have no effect, they usually pick on someone else.

A young woman with Tourette Syndrome describes how she came to terms with negative reactions:

> Granted there are people you encounter who are limited, and they seem to focus only on the tics. In such cases, all you can do is accept that they are not people with whom you are likely to become close. [As] an older man with TS [once] said, "I've finally come to a point in my life where I can no longer be bothered with people who reject me because of my symptoms."[14]

Even young people with severe TS symptoms often adjust remarkably well over time. A case in point is that of fourteen-year-old Lauren, who at eleven years of age found that having Tourette Syndrome made her life difficult both at home and in school. Fortunately, she's now doing quite well at a special high school that she describes as being "for kids with, you know, problems, like other kids with Tourette's." There, in an accepting, supportive atmosphere, Lauren takes the same courses offered in any high school—including shop. As part of a school-sponsored work-study program, she is employed part-time in a clothing store.

Part of Lauren's success may have grown out of her genuine acceptance of herself. She remarks:

> There's just a few kids that say I look for attention. . . . And it's gotten to the point where if you have nothing nice to say to me, leave me alone. I am who I am. You are who you are. . . . There are followers, there are leaders, and there are people who walk beside you. I didn't want to be a follower and I didn't want to be a leader. I want to be myself. Therefore, I am walking beside people. If you want to walk beside me, you can. And if you want to walk away, you can.[15]

chapter 4

Tourette Syndrome in the Spotlight

THE SUCCESS OF PROMINENT ATHLETES WITH TOURETTE Syndrome has greatly helped to dispel misconceptions about the disorder and raise awareness of it. The broad range of sports participated in by individuals with Tourette Syndrome is impressive—encompassing everything from Ping-Pong to mountain climbing. And the ability of these people to perform at a high level despite the disorder shows that Tourette Syndrome need not dampen the ambitions of young athletes. In fact, many researchers speculate that Tourette Syndrome allows some athletes to execute especially quick, rhythmic, and well-coordinated moves on a court or field. This is the finding of the well-respected neurologist Oliver Sacks, who writes, "This is not the case with everyone, but there is certainly a form of Tourette's in which extremely quick movements are symptomatic." Sack's extensive research with a Canadian karate expert who has Tourette Syndrome revealed that this athlete's movements were more than three times faster than average without any notable decrease in accuracy or precision. "He was not slowed down by his tics as they occurred but made immediate adjustments," Sacks observes. "This seems to be a sort of plus of Tourette's especially, I would think, for a basketball player."[1]

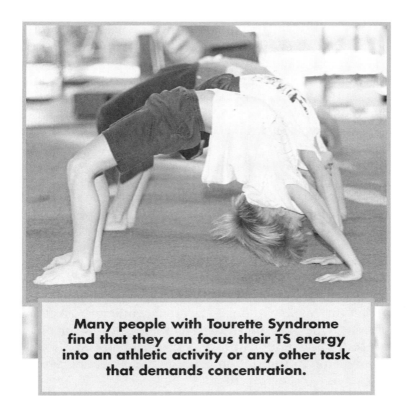

Many people with Tourette Syndrome find that they can focus their TS energy into an athletic activity or any other task that demands concentration.

MAHMOUD ABDUL-RAUF

One exceptional basketball player with Tourette Syndrome is Mahmoud Abdul-Rauf (formerly Chris Jackson), who grew up in Gulfport, Mississippi. Having Tourette Syndrome as a youth was tough for the now accomplished athlete. He recalls standing in the school yard unable to complete a basketball workout because the sound of the ball swishing through the net distracted him. It was even hard for him to leave home on time some mornings because it could take him fifteen minutes to tie his shoes until they felt just right to him. That same obsessive need for perfection was evident in his

41

classroom work. "In school, I'd have a hard time reading because I'd read the same sentence over and over," Abdul-Rauf recalls. "Each sentence had to come from my mind exactly right, and then it has to come off my lips right when I say it out loud, and I have to get the meaning right. When I was a kid trying to study, I'd spend an hour sometimes getting just one sentence perfect."[2]

Sensing that something was wrong, his mother took him to a doctor who was of little help. "He told me I had habits," Abdul-Rauf remembers. "I was young then and I didn't know better, so I figured, OK, I have habits. But I could have told him that going in."[3] He was not correctly diagnosed until his junior year in high school.

There is speculation that it is the precise combination of his drive for perfection, his natural athletic ability, and the disappearance of his TS symptoms when focused on a play that makes Abdul-Rauf an exceptional basketball player. "One sees that phenomenon with all forms of concentration among Tourettics," Sacks notes. "In the moment of concentration with a task at hand, people just seem to come together."[4]

Abdul-Rauf certainly excelled as a basketball star when he played on his college team at Louisiana State University. He set three NCAA records for freshmen and awed spectators when he scored 55 points in a game against Mississippi State University. The following year, as a sophomore, he won Player of the Year honors for the second year in a row, outdoing the now famous basketball player Shaquille O'Neal, who was a college teammate.

It has sometimes been reported that while in college, Abdul-Rauf was anxious to be drafted quickly by an NBA team because he thought his playing ability might deteriorate due to TS. This isn't so. His true motivation grew out of his desire to help his mother. At that time, she often had only water and eggs in her refrigerator and lived in such a shabby dwelling that one day the kitchen

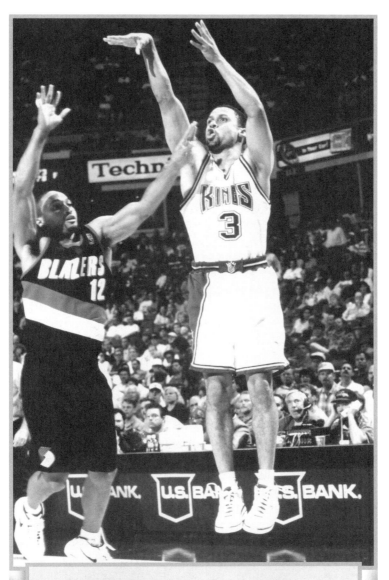

Mahmoud Abdul-Rauf has not let Tourette Syndrome stand in the way of his professional basketball career.

sink fell off the wall and crashed onto the floor. "That's when I realized she couldn't live like that anymore," Abdul-Rauf recalls. "That's when I resolved to get her the money so she wouldn't have to."[5]

Although Abdul-Rauf was signed by the Denver Nuggets after his sophomore year, his first two seasons were undistinguished. In his third season, however, he averaged 19.2 points a game and was named the league's Most Improved Player. That summer he visited Mecca, Saudi Arabia, and legally changed his name from Chris Jackson to Mahmoud Abdul-Rauf as part of his conversion to the Muslim faith. By the time the next basketball season rolled around he was considered an NBA All-Star.

Since then, Abdul-Rauf has been traded to the Sacramento Kings. His game, like that of any other professional athlete, has had its ups and downs. His devotion to Islam, however, has remained constant, and he believes he was given TS to test his faith. He says, "God has given me, through his blessing, Tourette's, and he has given me basketball and Islam to cope with Tourette's. Through basketball, I get a little peace. And through Islam, I get total peace."[6]

Fortunately, by the time Abdul-Rauf was ready to become a professional athlete, the sports world had learned about Tourette Syndrome through the well-publicized case of Jim Eisenreich, an outstanding baseball player with TS. In fact, when the Denver Nuggets first considered drafting Abdul-Rauf, a team official called Eisenreich to find out more about the disorder and how it might affect a rookie player on the court. "They asked me how it would affect him emotionally and physically, how the fans would react, how to tell them about it, [and] how [Abdul-Rauf] would be accepted," notes Eisenreich. "I knew he was one of the best basketball players in the country, and I told them everything would be fine."[7]

JIM EISENREICH

When Jim Eisenreich broke into major-league baseball in 1982, the sports world was still generally unaware of Tourette Syndrome. To make matters worse, Eisenreich hadn't even been diagnosed yet. Eisenreich's tics first surfaced while he was in grade school in St. Cloud, Minnesota. His father, concerned about the boy's health, took his son to a local doctor who was unable to arrive at a diagnosis. Young Eisenreich was taken for psychiatric evaluations, but as far as he knows no one knew what was wrong.

Yet the problem loomed large in Eisenreich's life. "I could never sit still for more than two to three minutes," Eisenreich remembers. "I used to get up and ask to go to the bathroom and do my tics. If I was at church, I'd walk out and come back when everyone was standing. But if I had to sit there, it was tough."[8]

Despite his untreated symptoms, Eisenreich's superior ability in baseball came through. A friend from Eisenreich's childhood who is now a professional baseball coach perhaps put it best when he remarked, "He always had tics and jerks but nobody ever said anything about it. Nobody wanted to mess him up. He was doing fine. Fortunately, most of his tics came while he was in the outfield or on the bench rather than when he was up at bat." But while Jim Eisenreich's teammates accepted him because of his winning ability on the field, this was not always true of opposing players. Eisenreich describes what playing Little League ball was like for him:

> When I was in Little League the kids on the other team would call me all sorts of names. I'd be breathing in and snorting, making all kinds of movements and the normal things that you do in Tourette Syndrome. They'd heckle me and give me a really bad time about it. I didn't like it but it never

really bothered me. I was a better player than they were.[9]

Even though Eisenreich seemed able to handle the ridicule, he saw that it affected other members of his family. "I think it made my Dad feel worse than me," he says. "He came up and asked me why I did it. Why was I making those faces? I started crying and said, 'I can't help it, I'm not trying to do it.'"[10]

Eisenreich's athletic ability also helped him overcome any unkind teasing or remarks when he went to St. Cloud State University and played baseball there. "The symptoms were present in college—the guttural sounds and shakes," comments Eisenreich's college teammate Bob Heyman, who later became a scout for the Kansas City Royals. "We just kind of accepted it. This was Jim Eisenreich. And it never affected his baseball. From Little League through college, Eisenreich would hum in the dugout to try to suppress the twitching. Never did he take himself out of a game, despite the taunts he heard from opposing players and fans."[11]

These sentiments are echoed by Dennis Lorsung, Eisenreich's college baseball coach. Lorsung explains that while he and Eisenreich's teammates certainly noticed the young man's unusual behavior, they chose to ignore it. "Jim was always making some sort of weird noise or movement out there in the field. At first the other outfielders noticed, but after a while they realized that it was just Jim."[12]

Things looked bright for Eisenreich at the start of his rookie year with the Minnesota Twins in 1982. Former Twins president Calvin Griffith had referred to Eisenreich as the finest ballplayer to come up through the team's farm system and predicted that the young player would become "a superstar and a millionaire in three years." But before long, the dreams for Eisenreich's future began to crumble. One day, while standing in center field in a game against Milwaukee, he began to

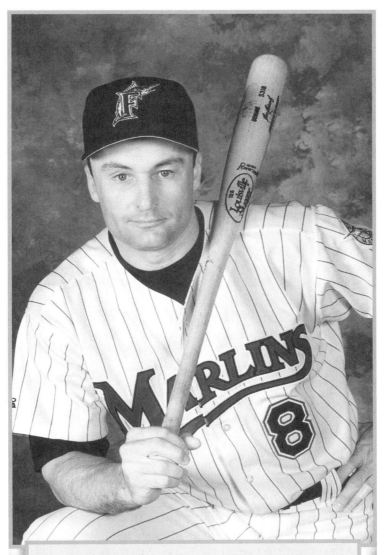

Jim Eisenreich's public triumph over Tourette Syndrome has raised awareness of the disorder and been an inspiration to people with and without TS.

twitch convulsively. Moments later, he felt unable to breathe and left the field. The same thing happened the following two evenings in front of more than 20,000 fans.

When the team went East to play a three-game series against Boston, the local fans had already heard about what happened on the field the week before. In Boston, on May 4, Eisenreich's tics resurfaced while he was on the field, and he began to hyperventilate. Once again, unable to continue playing, he left the field. To his team's disappointment, the scene repeated itself the next night with Eisenreich leaving the field even earlier. Days later, on May 7, Eisenreich wasn't able to stay in the game when his team played the Milwaukee Brewers. Feeling as though he was unable to expel the air from his lungs, he ran into the visitors' clubhouse yelling, "I can't breathe."

Eisenreich was taken to Mount Sinai Medical Center in downtown Milwaukee, where he was seen in the emergency room and given sedatives. Rather than being admitted to the hospital, Eisenreich was allowed to return to his hotel room where he remained while his teammates completed the games scheduled for the Twins' Milwaukee road trip. "This has always happened to me," he later said of the tics. "It just got really bad when I was with the Twins. I don't know why. Usually when I was in a situation like that—stuck on my breathing—it would always end before I got too hyped up. I could control it."[13]

The sports world was unfamiliar with Tourette Syndrome, and Eisenreich still hadn't been diagnosed. Many people assumed that the Minnesota Twins' would-be star rookie had psychiatric problems. Despite his natural playing ability, the team's management and Eisenreich's teammates believed that he was just unable to handle the stress of big-league baseball.

Dr. Leonard Michienzi, the Minnesota Twins team doctor, felt certain that Jim Eisenreich was suffering from "major-league stage fright" combined with agoraphobia (a fear of open or public places). He persisted in believing this even after the young player was finally diagnosed with Tourette Syndrome by Dr. Faruk Abuzzahab, an expert on the disorder. Abuzzahab's diagnosis was backed up by Dr. Arthur Shapiro, director of the Tourette and Tic Laboratory and Clinic of the Mount Sinai School of Medicine in New York City. "If Abuzzahab diagnosed him as having Tourette, he probably has it," Shapiro declared.[14]

The Minnesota Twins' view of Eisenreich's disorder as psychological rather than neurological worsened the situation for the young player. There were insinuations that anyone who couldn't handle the pressure didn't belong in major-league baseball. Some suggested that Eisenreich ought to stop hiding behind the TS diagnosis and own up to his "real" problems. Dr. Abuzzahab summed up the Twins' viewpoint when he noted, "He's [Eisenreich] a small-town boy. The Twins' doctor thought the limelight and attention aggravated his condition."[15]

In any case, after two weeks on the disabled list in 1982, Eisenreich agreed to take a drug for anxiety prescribed by the Twins' doctor. At first things went well, but before long the medication caused drowsiness that affected his play. "I was beat, physically tired," Eisenreich remembers. "I was taking a lot of medication."[16] Three weeks later, he was back on the disabled list.

In 1983, Eisenreich did well at spring training, batting .400 in the exhibition season. But the following week, he felt the problem returning and backed off the idea of playing. Eisenreich spent the remainder of the season seeing psychiatrists and hypnotists recommended by the Twins. The Twins had Eisenreich back at spring training in 1984, and he was the leadoff player in the season's opening game against Detroit. He played in twelve games before the growing tension between

Eisenreich and Twins' physician Michienzi finally erupted.

Michienzi had learned that Eisenreich had been secretly taking medication for Tourette Syndrome prescribed by his family doctor. Fearing that the drugs might weaken his performance, the Twins' management refused to tolerate Eisenreich receiving outside medical care. He was told to take the pills for anxiety that Michienzi had prescribed for him and to discontinue his TS medication. If he refused to comply, he would be sent down to the Twins' minor-league team. It was a no-win situation for Eisenreich, who didn't see the point of taking medication for a condition he didn't have while giving up his drugs for TS, which were helping. After he refused to go to the minors, he was given a final option of taking a year's salary and retiring. Eisenreich left the team and never played for the Twins again.

Eisenreich returned to major-league baseball in 1987 as a member of the Kansas City Royals. He has no ill will against the Minnesota Twins, realizing that they never really understood Tourette Syndrome. However, one can't help but wonder how the Twins felt when, in a game against the Kansas City Royals, Jim Eisenreich beat them by driving in the winning run. It's further reported that following Eisenreich's first home run for the Royals, the fans' cheered and applauded until Eisenreich stepped out of the dugout to acknowledge their praise. One sportswriter described the scene this way, "The Royals fans have a tremendous amount of respect and admiration for his courage and strength, not to mention his talent. They just love him. The Twins must be kicking themselves that they gave up on him because this guy never gave up on himself."[17]

As a member of the Royals for six years, Jim Eisenreich had several outstanding seasons. Jim Eisenreich then played successfully for the Philadelphia Phillies, where he was one of the city's best-loved players. In 1997, he was traded to the Florida Marlins and contributed to the team's World Series victory by batting .500 during the seven-game series. Eisenreich's success has been an inspiration to people with or without Tourette Syndrome. The extensive media coverage he has received has allowed people to see that TS need not be a disability.

Eisenreich has been a dedicated spokesman for the TS cause, and in 1996 he established the Jim Eisenreich Foundation for children who suffer from Tourette Syndrome. When asked what advice he has for young people diagnosed with TS, Jim Eisenreich has said, "Well, I suppose the only thing I would say is just do whatever you want to do. That's what I've always done. Don't let anything hold you back from it. . . . You can do anything you want to. You can't let other people bother you."[18] Jim Eisenreich's successful major-league baseball career serves as proof of his words.

chapter 5

Success

WHILE MANY YOUNG PEOPLE WITH TOURETTE SYNDROME HAVE struggled with their symptoms, countless success stories balance the picture. Sixth-grade spelling champion Patrick Murphy of Riddle, Oregon, is a great example. Patrick triumphed over the competition at district-level spelling bees to win an award at a county event. In some cases, Patrick competed against seventh- and eighth-graders and won. Having TS has not stopped this dynamic young person from being involved in other activities as well. Patrick is in a school singing group, a chess club, and is active in various church programs.

Young people with TS often excel athletically, too. Seventeen-year-old Chris Blaubery of New York ran in the Long Island marathon, completing the race in an impressive four hours and fifty-three minutes. Middle-school student Joseph Shortt of Long Island, New York, has become something of a sports hero in his hometown for his ability on the basketball court. According to the Tourette Syndrome Association's newsletter, Joseph's honors include being voted Most Valuable Player. Shortt, who's also an outstanding baseball player, was a starting pitcher and had the highest batting average on the team.

Adults with TS have also been exceedingly successful. In fact, there are few challenges people with TS haven't taken on and conquered. There are writers, chemists, mathematicians, clergy, musicians, computer programmers, mechanics, psychologists, social workers, ecologists, teachers, doctors, and athletes with Tourette Syndrome whose symptoms vary from mild to severe.

Is there anything someone with Tourette Syndrome cannot do? Are there professions or pastimes off limits to a person with the disorder because the symptoms might interfere with what needs to be done? "Some things one might think, would be completely out of the question," notes neurologist Oliver Sacks, who has extensively studied Tourette Syndrome. "Above all, perhaps, the intricate, precise, and steady work of a surgeon. This would have been my own belief not so long ago. But now, improbably, I know five surgeons with Tourette's."[1]

DR. CARL BENNETT

Among these surgeons is Dr. Carl Bennett. Oliver Sacks first met Bennett at a medical conference on Tourette Syndrome in Boston. Bennett appeared dignified, conservatively dressed, and ordinary enough. But periodically, Sacks writes, "He suddenly lunged or reached for the ground or jumped or jerked." After speaking to him for a time, Bennett invited Sacks to his hometown so he'd have an opportunity to observe a surgeon with Tourette Syndrome in both a work and social environment. Sacks, a longtime student of the subtler effects of Tourette Syndrome, eagerly took him up on the offer.

Dr. Bennett's TS had started when he was a seven-year-old boy living with his family in Toronto, Canada. "I wore glasses, I had bands on my teeth and I twitched," describes Bennett. "I kept my distance. I was a loner. . . . I never had friends calling all the time. . . . I'd go for long hikes by myself."[2]

Apparently, being on his own much of the time toughened Bennett, making him both resourceful and independent. This later helped him deal with the exhausting course load and work schedule in medical school. Having TS made medical school especially difficult for Bennett because there was quite a bit of reading to do and his TS interfered with that. "I'd have to read each line many times," he remembers. "I'd have to line up each paragraph to get all four corners symmetrically in my visual field."[3] Although this process slowed Bennett's reading, by the time he graduated he practically knew his medical texts by heart, affording him a range of knowledge few other physicians could boast of.

After medical school, Bennett developed an expertise in polar medicine while working in far northwestern Canada. Following his marriage, he and his new wife took a trip around the world. Bennett had an opportunity to realize his childhood dream of climbing Mount Kilimanjaro.

When Carl Bennett first began his medical practice in Branford (a town in western Canada), he was looked upon suspiciously as a surgeon who twitches. However, he soon proved his ability in the operating room, and before long his practice grew. Before Bennett got to know someone well, he would try to conceal or downplay his tics. For example, when he first came to the Branford hospital, he tried to repress his urges to hop and skip down the corridors. But after the staff became used to Bennett, he was able to give in to the urge without anyone giving him a second glance.

During his visit with Bennett at the hospital, Dr. Sacks was especially struck by a scene in the doctors' lounge. "The conversations in the room were like those of any hospital," Sacks explains. "Bennett, himself, lying half-curled on the floor, kicking and thrusting one foot in the air described an unusual case. . . . His colleagues listened attentively. The abnormality of the behavior and the complete normality of the discourse formed an extraordinary contrast. There was something bizarre about the whole scene, but it was evidently so common . . . as to no longer attract the slightest notice. But an outsider seeing it would have been stunned."[4]

Perhaps even more amazing was Dr. Bennett in the operating room. His TS symptoms were obvious, but they never interfered with his precise surgical skill. As Oliver Sacks relates, "What I saw in the outpatient clinic was magnified [in the operating room]: constant dartings and reachings with the hands, almost but never quite touching his unscrubbed, unsterile shoulder, . . . sudden lungings and touching of his colleagues with his feet; and a barrage of vocalizations—Hooty-hooo! Hooty-hooo!—suggestive of a huge owl."[5]

Yet as soon as Bennett made the first incision with his surgical knife, there was no sign of any sort of tic. Throughout the complex surgery, Bennett's movements were smooth, quick, and precise. The entire two-and-a-half-hour operation was successfully completed without the slightest hint of TS. Bennett does not have to concentrate on holding back tics while operating—the impulses just seem to disappear. "His whole identity at such times is that of a surgeon at work," Sacks remarks. "And his entire psychic and neural organization becomes aligned with this, becomes active, focused, at ease, un-Tourettic."[6] If Bennett's concentration is broken, perhaps to review an X ray during the surgery, the tics momentarily return. Once he starts operating again, however, the tics are gone. "It's like a miracle," one of his colleagues remarked. "The way the Tourette's disappears." Although it may seem so, Bennett's TS has not actually vanished. According to Oliver Sacks, the Tourette's energy is "organized and mastered, its force all coordinated in the act of performance."[7]

TOURETTE SYNDROME AND CREATIVITY

Many talented actors, musicians, writers, and artists have Tourette Syndrome. Peter Antico, an actor with Tourette Syndrome, has appeared in films such as *Lethal*

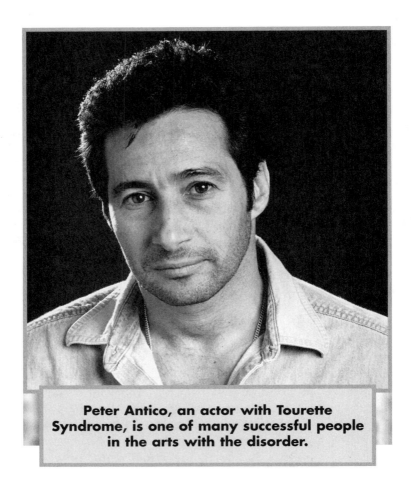

Peter Antico, an actor with Tourette Syndrome, is one of many successful people in the arts with the disorder.

Weapon 3 with Mel Gibson and *29th Street* with Danny Aiello. He has long been determined not to let TS stop him from being who he wants to be. As a child, his TS was fairly severe; his symptoms included shoulder tics, cursing, and what he's described as "a lot of mental tics . . . like 25 different thoughts coming into your head at the same time."

However, Antico found that when he became extremely involved or focused on a particular task, his TS symptoms temporarily faded out. In high school, this enabled him to excel at pole-vaulting—among the most technical events in track and field. Antico also played college baseball. His college coach used to tell him, "Pete, every time you're up at the plate, you don't move a muscle, and you have great focus."[8]

David Aldrige, a jazz musician, finds that his TS symptoms were not always readily distinguishable from his musical talent. Aldrige writes, "Rhythm and Tourette Syndrome have been intertwined from the first day I found that drumming on a table could mask my jerky hand, leg and neck movements. . . . [It] could harness my unbounding [Tourette's] energy directing it into an orderly flow." He adds that he would sometimes ride his own "Tourettic stream . . . so the roller-coaster ride of Tourette's could be transformed."[9]

Some medical scholars argue that even the brilliant musician Mozart may have had Tourette Syndrome. There is evidence that Mozart had very noticeable tics. At least fourteen firsthand witnesses noted Mozart's "motor or vocal peculiarities." This was written of him in 1793:

> [Mozart's] features would alter from one instant to another, yet never revealing anything save the pleasure or the distress that he happened to feel in that immediate instant. . . . His body was perpetually in motion; he would play incessantly with his hands or tap restlessly with his feet.[10]

Apparently Mozart's tics became especially obvious to his sister-in-law and other family members at the opera. She described the "restless movements of his hands" and the continuous "movements of his lips" implying that he was unable to keep still during any part of the performance.

It is further thought that coprolalia was among Mozart's TS symptoms; he was known for obscene outbursts that could occur at any time without warning.

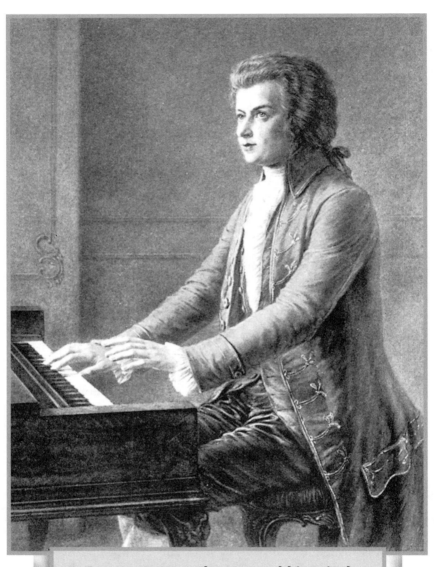

Experts suspect that several historical
figures may have had Tourette Syndrome.
Mozart is one of the most
prominent of these.

"He [Mozart] took delight [in] . . . these vulgar [rantings]," an actor and friend once wrote of him.[11]

One successful author with TS developed two distinctly different styles of writing. When writing formal and informative reviews and essays, he keeps his TS urges tightly in check. In the other mode, "he lets himself go and, at great speed, writes huge meandering, fantastical (and often coprolalic) novels, in which he gives his Tourettic fancies full rein."[12]

Novelist Kurt Tidmore, who has had TS for as long as he can remember, also claims that it helps with his writing:

> On a good day, the words pour out of me in something I can only liken to a verbal hallucination. I work at them with a kind of athletic improvisation, like a basketball star driving into the lane for a layup. If I'm not talking, I'm typing as fast as I can to keep up with the flow. That's another place Tourette's helps. Touretters have great reflexes—I can type nearly a hundred words a minute. I also play the piano, the trombone, the saxophone and the recorder, and I can whistle like a bird. Touretters are nearly always musical.[13]

Although some individuals with Tourette Syndrome have been able to mold and positively channel the intense energy generated by their disorder, it is important not to glamorize a neurological problem that can sometimes be extremely distressful. Even the creative Tourettic drive can be difficult to handle. Kurt Tidmore refers to this drive as "wildness." "That's the word for it," he explains. "It's something untamed—[something] that helps me write stories and play music also leads me into rages that flare up as quickly as a gasoline fire. They come like that and then they are gone, leaving the tamer part of me to pick up the pieces."[14]

Dr. Carl Bennett is also aware that his Tourettic energy always resides just beneath the surface. He feels there is only a "thin line of control between the person with TS . . . [and] that raging storm." He explains, "One can see the charming things, the funny things . . . but there's also that dark side. . . . You have to fight it all your life."[15]

MORE THAN JUST TICS

Many people feel that the experience of having Tourette Syndrome often plays a part in shaping the personalities of those with the disorder. Remember, though, that it is not the only part. "I can't remember when I didn't make sounds or have to do my rituals," one young woman with Tourette Syndrome relates. "I thought this 'crazy' girl was the only person I was. After all, practically everything that ever happened to me—from medical attention, therapy, special placements in school to hospitalizations—stemmed from my having TS. I walked around thinking 'I am TS.' Only in the last few years have I been thinking there's a real personality in here somewhere—that there's more to me than tics."[16]

Source Notes

Chapter 1

1. Sandra Blakeslee, "Studies Pinpoint Region of Brain Implicated in Tourette Syndrome," *New York Times,* September 17, 1996, C3.
2. ABC News *20/20,* July 31, 1992, transcript #1232, 12.
3. Tracy Haerle, *Children with Tourette Syndrome: A Parent's Guide* (Rockville, MD: Woodbine House, 1992), 15.
4. Blakeslee.
5. *20/20* transcript #1232, 13.
6. Ibid.
7. Ibid.

Chapter 2

1. Blakeslee.
2. National Institute of Mental Health, "Obsessive Compulsive Disorder" (pamphlet), September 1994, 16.
3. Haerle, 23.
4. Haerle, 67.

Chapter 3

1. Mark Phillips, "Possessed," *New York Times Magazine,* July 4, 1993, 8.
2. Ibid.
3. Ibid.
4. *Maury Povich Show,* "Children with Tourette," December 26, 1995, transcript.
5. Haerle, 25.

6. Phillips.
7. *Povich.*
8. Ibid.
9. Ibid.
10. Ibid.
11. Haerle, 51.
12. Haerle, 109.
13. Jared Berstein, *Coping with TS in Early Adulthood* (New York: Tourette Syndrome Association, 1997), 5.
14. Ibid.
15. *Povich.*

Chapter 4

1. Bruce Schoenfeld, "A Separate Peace," *Sporting News,* February 14, 1994, 29.
2. Ibid.
3. Ibid., 30.
4. Ibid.
5. Ibid.
6. Ibid., 31.
7. Ibid.
8. Jeff Shear, "When Anxiety Comes to Bat," *New York Times Magazine,* March 8, 1987, 75.
9. Richard Demak, "Fighting the Enemy Within," *Sports Illustrated,* June 22, 1987, 43.
10. Alan Levitt, "Jim Eisenreich: Back to the Dream," Tourette Syndrome Association, 1987, 1.
11. Demak, 42.

12. Shear, 74.
13. Demak, 41.
14. Ibid., 42.
15. Ibid.
16. Shear, 76.
17. Levitt, 3.
18. Ibid., 4.

Chapter 5

1. Oliver Sacks, "A Surgeon's Life," *New Yorker*, March 16, 1992, 85.
2. Ibid., 87.
3. Ibid., 88.
4. Ibid., 89.
5. Ibid., 91.
6. Ibid., 92.
7. Oliver Sacks, "Tourette Syndrome and Creativity," *British Medical Journal*, 19–26 December, 1992, 1516.
8. Sacks, "Tourette Syndrome and Creativity," 1515.
9. Povich.
10. Benjamin Simkin, "Mozart's Scatological Disorder," *British Medical Journal*, 19–26 December, 1992, 1564.
11. Ibid.
12. Sacks, "Tourette Syndrome and Creativity," 1515.
13. Kurt Tidmore, "The Twitch," *Natural Health*, May–June 1995, 176.
14. Ibid.
15. Sacks, "A Surgeon's Life," 43.
16. Berstein, 5.

For More Information

BOOKS

Bruun, Ruth Dowling. *A Mind of Its Own: Tourette's Syndrome: A Story and a Guide*. New York: Oxford University Press, 1994.

Fowler, Rick. *The Unwelcome Companion: An Insider's View of Tourette Syndrome*. Cashiers, NC: Silver Run Publications, 1996.

Hughes, Susan. *Ryan: A Mother's Story of Her Hyperactive/Tourette Syndrome Child*. Duarte, CA: Hope Press, 1990.

Shimberg, Elaine Fantle. *Living with Tourette Syndrome*. New York: Simon & Schuster, 1995.

INTERNET RESOURCES

Articles, Commentaries & Information Papers
http://www.ccn.cs.dal.ca/ Health/Tourette/info/ commentaries.html
Online articles on TS from the Nova Scotia Tourette Syndrome Information Site

Facts about Tourette Syndrome
http://www.geocities.com/ Athens/Forum/6903/tourette. html
This site offers a well-organized description of the disorder. It also includes a list of relevant links.

Gilles De La Tourette Syndrome
http://www3.ncbi.nlm.nih. gov/htbin-post/Omim/ dispmim?137580
Very detailed—though technical—information about TS from the National Institutes of Health.

Hope Press
http://www.infoboard.com/ tourette/
Hope Press is a publisher that specializes in books on Tourette Syndrome and ADHD. This site provides a list of their publications including summaries, reviews, and ordering information.

Internet Mental Health
http://www.mentalhealth. com/fr20.html
This site offers excellent information on all kinds of mental and neurological disorders including Tourette Syndrome.

National Institute of Neurological Disorders and Stroke Tourette Syndrome Page
http://www.ninds.nih.gov/ healinfo/disorder/tourette/ tourette.htm
Facts about TS from a division of

the National Institutes of Health. See p. 65 for this organization's address.

Tourette Syndrome Association
http://tsa.mgh.harvard.edu/
Offers lots of detailed information about TS including a list of answers to frequently asked questions. Includes a directory of Tourette Syndrome Association chapters throughout the United States. See the next column for more information about this organization.

What Makes Tics Tick? Clues Found in Tourette Twins' Caudates
http://www.nimh.nih.gov/ events/prtouret.htm
This is a summary of the study conducted by the National Institute of Mental Health on pairs of identical twins with Tourette Syndrome. This study, mentioned on pp. 16–17, leads scientists to believe that tics associated with TS are influenced by the way dopamine is processed in the brain.

ORGANIZATIONS

A number of public and private agencies can be helpful in providing information on the educational, legal, health-care and residential rights and needs of people with TS and other disorders. A partial listing is provided here.

Tourette Syndrome Association, Inc.
National Headquarters
42–40 Bell Boulevard
Bayside, New York 11361–9596
(718) 224–2999;
(800) 237–0717
The Tourette Syndrome Association, Inc., is a national voluntary nonprofit organization with local chapters throughout the country. The group offers a wide range of information and resources for individuals with TS and their families. Call the national headquarters for the current addresses and telephone numbers of local chapters.

Other National Organizations

American Association of University Affiliated Programs for Persons with Developmental Disabilities (AAUAP)
860 Fenton Street, Suite 410
Silver Springs, MD 20910
(301) 588–8252

Association for the Care Of Children's Health (ACCH)
7910 Woodmount Avenue, Suite 300
Bethesda, MD 20814
(301) 654–6549

Children and Adults With Attention Deficit Disorders (CH.A.D.D.)
499 Northwest 70th Avenue, Suite 101

Plantation, Florida 33317
(800) 233–4050;
(954) 587–4599 (Fax)

City Of Hope National Medical
  Center
Department of Medical Genetics
Duarte, CA 91010
(818) 359–8111, ext. 2631

Disability Rights Education and
  Defense Fund, Inc.
2212 Sixth Street
Berkeley, CA 94710
(415) 644–2555

Learning Disabilities Association
  of America (LDAA)
4156 Library Road
Pittsburgh, PA 15234
(412) 340–1515

National Association of
  Protection and Advocacy
  Systems
900 2nd Street, NE, Suite 211
Washington, DC 20002
(202) 408–9514

National Center for Hyperactive
  Children
5535 Balboa Boulevard,
  Suite 215
Encino, CA 91316
(818) 986–0514; (818) 780–9819

National Center for Youth with
  Disabilities
University of Minnesota
Box 721–UMHC
Harvard Street at East River Road
Minneapolis, MN 55455

(612) 626–2825;
(800) 333–NCYD

National Institute of Neurological
  Disorders and Stroke (NINDS)
National Institutes of Health
9000 Rockville Pike
Bethesda, MD 20892
(301) 496–5751

National Organization for Rare
  Disorders (NORD)
P.O. Box 8923
New Fairfield, CT 06812
(203) 746–6518; (800) 999–6673

National Organization on
  Disability (NOD)
910 16th Street, NW, Suite 600
Washington, DC 20006
(202) 293–5960;
(800) 248–ABLE

Obsessive Compulsive
  Foundation
P.O. Box 9673
New Haven, CT 06535
(203) 772–0565

U.S. Department of Education Office of Civil Rights Chapters

Region I (Connecticut, Maine,
  Massachusetts, New
  Hampshire, Rhode Island,
  Vermont):
U. S. Department of Education
Office for Civil Rights
J. W. McCormack Post Office and
  Courthouse Building, Room
  222, 01–0061
Boston, MA 02109–4557

(617) 223–9662;
(617) 223–9565 (TDD)

Region II (New Jersey, New York, Puerto Rico, Virgin Islands):
U.S. Department of Education
Office for Civil Rights
26 Federal Plaza, 33rd Floor, Room 330130, 02–1010
New York, NY 10278–0082
(212) 264–4633;
(212) 264–9464 (TDD)

Region III (Delaware, District of Columbia, Maryland,
Pennsylvania, Virginia, West Virginia):
U.S. Department of Education
Office for Civil Rights
3535 Market Street, Room 6300, 03–2010
Philadelphia, PA 19104–3326
(215) 596–6772;
(215) 596–6794 (TDD)

Region IV (Alabama, Florida, Georgia, Kentucky, Mississippi, North
Carolina, South Carolina, Tennessee):
U.S. Department of Education
Office for Civil Rights
101 Marietta Tower, 27th Floor, Suite 2702
P.O. Box 1705, 04–3010
Atlanta, GA 30310–1705
(404) 331–2954;
(404) 331–7816 (TDD)

Region V (Illinois, Indiana, Michigan, Minnesota, Ohio, Wisconsin):
U.S. Department of Education

Office for Civil Rights
401 South State Street, Room 700C, 05–4010
Chicago, IL 60606–1202
(312) 886–3456;
(312) 353–2541 (TDD)

Region VI (Arkansas, Louisiana, New Mexico, Oklahoma, Texas):
U.S. Department of Education
Office for Civil Rights
1200 Main Tower Building, Suite 2260, 06–5010
Dallas, TX 75202–9998
(214) 767–3959;
(214) 767–3639 (TDD)

Region VII (Iowa, Kansas, Missouri, Nebraska):
U.S. Department of Education
Office for Civil Rights
10220 North Executive Hills Boulevard,
8th Floor
P.O. Box 901381, 07–6010
Kansas City, MO 64190–1381
(816) 891–8026

Region VIII (Colorado, Montana, North Dakota,
South Dakota, Utah, Wyoming)
U.S. Department of Education
Office for Civil Rights
Federal Office Building
1961 Stout Street, Room 342, 08–7010
Denver, CO 80294–3608
(303) 884–5695;
(303) 884–3417 (TDD)

Region IX (Arizona, California, Hawaii, Nevada, Guam, Trust

Territory of Pacific Islands,
American Samoa):
U.S. Department of Education
Office for Civil Rights
221 Main Street, 10th Floor,
Suite 1020, 09–8010
San Francisco, CA 94105–1925
(415) 227–8040;
(415) 227–8124 (TDD)

Region X (Alaska, Idaho, Oregon,
Washington):
U.S. Department of Education
Office for Civil Rights
915 Second Avenue, Room 3310,
10–9010
Seattle, WA 98174–1099
(206) 442–1636;
(206) 442–4542 (TDD)

Local Organizations
(by State)

Alabama
Alabama Association for Children
and Adults
with Learning Disabilities
(ACLD)
P.O. Box 11588
Montgomery, AL 36111
(205) 277–9151

Department of Mental Health
and Mental Retardation
200 Interstate Park Drive
Montgomery, AL 36193
(205) 271–9208

Sparks Center for Developmental
and Learning Disorders
University of Alabama at
Birmingham

1720 Seventh Avenue, South
Birmingham, AL 35233
(205) 934–5471

Special Education Action
Committee (SEAC)
P.O. Box 161274
Mobile, AL 36616–2274
(205) 478–1208;
(800) 222–7322 (in Alabama)

Alaska
Alaska Association for Children
and Adults with Learning
Disabilities (ACLD)
108 West Cook Avenue
Anchorage, AK 99051
(907) 279–1662

Office of Special Services
Department of Education
Pouch F
Juneau, AL 99811
(907) 465–2970

Division of Vocational
Rehabilitation
Department of Education
Pouch F. Mail Stop 0581
State Office Building.
Juneau, AK 99811
(907) 456–2814

Developmental Disabilities
Planning Council
600 University Avenue, Suite B
Fairbanks, AK 99709–3651
(907) 479–6507

Advocacy Services of Alaska
325 East Third Avenue,
2nd Floor
Anchorage, AK 99501

Arizona

Special Education
Department of Education
1535 West Jefferson
Phoenix, AS 85007-3280
(602) 542-3183

Rehabilitation Services Bureau
Department of Economic
  Security
1300 West Washington Street
Phoenix, AS 85007
(602) 524-3332

Division of Developmental
  Disabilities Department of
  Economic Security
P.O. Box 6123
Phoenix, AZ 85005
(602) 258-0419

Arkansas

Association for Children and
  Adults with Learning
  Disabilities (ACLD)
State Office
P. O. Box 7316
Little Rock, AR 72217
(501) 666-8777

Special Education Section
Department of Education
Education Building,
Room 105-C
Little Rock, AR 72201
(501) 682-4221

Special Education Section
  (Ages 3-5)
Department of Education
4 Capital Mall, Room 105-C
Little Rock, AR 72201
(501) 682-4222

Division of Rehabilitation
  Services
Department of Human Services
P.O. Box 3781
7th and Main Streets
Little Rock, AR 72203
(501) 682-6708

Governor's Developmental
  Disabilities Planning Council
4815 West Markham Street
Little Rock, AR 72201
(501) 661-2589

California

Tourette Syndrome Clinic
Department of Medical Genetics
City of Hope National Medical
  Center
Duarte, CA 91010
(818) 359-8111, ext. 2631;
(818) 357-7624

Association for Children and
  Adults with Learning
  Disabilities (ACLD)
State Office
17 Buena Vista Avenue
Mill Valley, CA 94941
(415) 383-5242

Special Education Division
California Department of
  Education
721 Capitol Mall
Sacramento, CA 94244-2720
(916) 323-4768

Department of Rehabilitation
Health and Welfare Agency
830 K Street Mall
Sacramento, CA 95814
(916) 445-3971

68

Department of Developmental
  Services
Health and Welfare Agency
1600 9th Street NW,
2nd Floor
Sacramento, CA 95814
(916) 323–3131

State Council on Developmental
  Disabilities
200 O Street, Room 100
Sacramento, CA 95814
(916) 322–8481

Center for Child Development
  and Developmental Disorders
University Affiliated Training
  Programs
Children's Hospital of
  Los Angeles
4650 Sunset Boulevard
Los Angeles, CA 90027
(213) 669–2151

Colorado

Colorado Association for
  Children with Learning
  Disabilities (ACLD)
1835 Cherry
Denver, CO 80220
(303) 973–3134

State Office ACLD
P.O. Box 32188
Aurora, CO 80041
(303) 973–3134

Special Education Services Unit
Department of Education
201 East Colfax Avenue
Denver, CO 80203
(303) 866–6694

Division of Rehabilitation
Department of Social Services
1575 Sherman Street,
4th Fl.
Denver, CO 80203
(303) 866–5196

Division for Developmental
  Disabilities
3824 West Princeton Circle
Denver, CO 80236
(303) 762–4560

Colorado Developmental
  Disabilities Council
777 Grant Street, Suite 410
Denver, CO 80203–3528
(303) 894–2345

Connecticut

Association for Children with
  Learning Disabilities (ACLD)
27 Brainard Road
West Hartford, CT 06117

ACLD State Office
139 North Main Street
Boatner Building
West Hartford, CT 06107
(860) 236–3953

Bureau of Special Education and
  Pupil Personnel Services
Department of Education
25 Industrial Park Road
Middletown, CT 06457
(860) 638–4265

Early Childhood Unit (Ages 3–5)
Division of Curriculum and
  Professional Development
Department of Education
P.O. Box 2219

Hartford, CT 06145
(860) 566–5670

Division of Rehabilitation
  Services
Board of Education
10 Griffin Road North
Windsor, CT 06195

Department of Children and
  Youth Services
170 Sigourney Street
Hartford, CT 06115
(860) 566–8614

Developmental Disabilities
  Council
90 Pitkin Street
East Hartford, CT 06108
(860) 725–3829

Connecticut's University
  Affiliated Program on
  Developmental Disabilities
991 Main Street
East Hartford, CT 06108
(860) 282–7050

Delaware
Delaware Association for
  Children with Learning
  Disabilities (ACLD)
177 East Sutton Pl.
Wilmington, DE 19810
(302) 994–0707

ACLD
State Office of New Castle
  County
P.O. Box 577
Bear, DE 19701
(302) 994–0707

Exceptional Children/Special
  Programs Division
Department of Public Instruction
P.O. Box 1402
Dover, DE 19903
(302) 739–5471

Division of Vocational
  Rehabilitation
Department of Labor
321 East 11th Street
Wilmington, DE 19801
(302) 577–2850

Developmental Disabilities
  Council
156 South State Street
P.O. Box 1401
Dover, DE 19903
(302) 736–4456

District of Columbia
District of Columbia Association
  for Children with Learning
  Disabilities (ACLD)
1648 NW Hobart Street
Washington, DC 29999
(202) 462–0495

ACLD State Office
P.O. Box 6350
Washington, DC 20015

Division of Special Education
D.C. Public Schools
10th and H Streets, NW
Washington, DC 20001
(202) 724–4018

Vocational Rehabilitation Services
  Administration
Department of Human Resources
605 G. Street, NW, No. 1101

Washington, DC 20001
(202) 727–3227

Child/Youth Services
  Administration
DC Commission on Mental
  Health Services
1120 19th Street, NW, No. 700
Washington, DC 20036
(202) 673–7784

Developmental Disabilities
  Planning Council
801 North Capitol, NE
Washington, DC 20001
(202) 724–5696

Florida
Florida ACLD
7016 North Donald Avenue
Tampa, FL 33614
(813) 637–8957

Bureau of Education for
  Exceptional Children
Department of Education
325 West Gaines Street, No. 614
Tallahassee, FL 32399
(904) 488–1570

Division of Vocational
  Rehabilitation
Department of Labor and
  Employment Security
1709–A Mahan Drive
Tallahassee, FL 32399
(904) 488–6210

Developmental Services Program
  Office
Department of Health and
  Rehabilitative Services
1311 Winewood Boulevard

Building 5, Room 215
Tallahassee, FL 32301
(904) 488–4257

Mental Health Services,
  Children's Program
Alcohol, Drug Abuse, and Mental
  Health Program Office
1317 Winewood Boulevard
Tallahassee, FL 32301
(904) 487–2415

Florida Developmental
  Disabilities Planning Council
820 East Park Avenue,
No. 1–100
Tallahassee, FL 32301
(904) 488–4180

Advocacy Center for Persons
  with Disabilities
2661 Executive Center Circle,
  West
Suite 100
Tallahassee, FL 32301
(904) 488–9071

Georgia
Georgia ACLD
3160 Northside Pkwy, NW
Atlanta, GA 30327
(404) 633–5332

ACLD State Office
P.O. Box 29492
Atlanta, GA 30359
(404) 656–2425

Program for Exceptional Students
Department of Education
1970 Twin Towers East
Atlanta, GA 30334
(404) 656–2425

Division of Rehabilitation
  Services
Department of Human Resources
878 Peachtree Street, NE,
Room 706
Atlanta, GA 30309
(404) 894–6670

Georgia Council on
  Developmental Disabilities
878 Peachtree Street, NE
Atlanta, GA 30309
(404) 894–5790

Georgia Advocacy Office, Inc.
Suite 811
1708 Peachtree Street, NW,
No. 505
Atlanta, GA 30309
(404) 885–1447; (800) 537–4538

University Affiliated Program of
  Georgia
570 Aderhold Hall
Athens, GA 30602
(404) 542–1685

Hawaii
Hawaii ACLD
1st Hawaiian Bank
P.O. Box 3200 Honolulu, HI
  96847
(808) 525–7098

Hawaii State Office ACLD
200 North Vineyard Boulevard
Suite 103
Honolulu, HI 96817
(808) 536–9684

Special Education Section
Department of Education
3430 Leahi Avenue

Honolulu, HI 96815
(808) 737–3720

Division of Vocational
  Rehabilitation
Department of Human Services
1000 Bishop Street, No. 615
Honolulu, HI 96813
(808) 548–4769

Child and Adolescent Mental
  Health Division
3627 Kilauea Avenue, Suite 101
Honolulu, HI 96816
(808) 548–3906

State Planning Council on
  Developmental Disabilities
501 Ala Moana Boulevard,
No. 200
Honolulu, HI 96813
(808) 548–8482

Protection and Advocacy Agency
1580 Makaloa Street, Suite 1060
Honolulu, HI 96814
(808) 949–2992

Special Parent Information
  Network
335 Merchant Street, Room 353
Honolulu, HI 96813
(808) 548–2648

Idaho
Idaho ACLD
4610–A Jackson Place
Mountain Home AFB, ID 83648
(208) 832–4218

Special Education Division
Department of Education
Len B. Jordan Building

650 West State Street
Boise, ID 83720–0001
(208) 334–3940

Division of Vocational
  Rehabilitation
State Board of Vocational
  Rehabilitation
650 West State Street
Boise, ID 83720
(208) 334–3390

Bureau of Developmental
  Disabilities
Division of Community
  Rehabilitation
Department of Health and
  Welfare
450 West State,
7th Floor
Boise, ID 83720
(208) 334–5531

Idaho State Council on
  Developmental Disabilities
280 North 8th Street,
No. 208
Boise, ID 83720
(208) 334–2178

Illinois
Illinois ACLD
19525 West Washington
Grayslake, IL 60030
(312) 223–6681, Ext. 220

Illinois ACLD
P.O. Box A–3239
Chicago, IL 60690
(312) 663–9535

ACLD State Office
400 East Sibley Boulevard

Room 111
Harvey, IL 60426
(708) 210–3532

Department of Special
  Education
State Board of Education
100 North First Street
Springfield, IL 62777
(217) 782–6601

Department of Rehabilitation
  Services
State Board of Vocational
  Rehabilitation
623 East Adams Street
P.O. Box 19429
Springfield, IL 62794

Department of Mental Health
  and Developmental Disabilities
402 Stratton Office Building
Springfield, IL 62706
(217) 782–7395

Institute for Juvenile Research
907 South Wolcott
Chicago, IL 60612
(312) 996–1733

University Affiliated Facility for
  Developmental Disabilities
University of Illinois at Chicago
1640 West Roosevelt Road
Chicago, IL 60608
(312) 413–1647

Coordinating Council for
  Handicapped Children
20 East Jackson Boulevard,
Room 900
Chicago, IL 60604
(312) 939–3513

73

Indiana

Indiana Association for Children
and Adults with Learning
Disabilities (ACLD)
7367 East 16th Street
Indianapolis, IN 46219
(317) 357–8268

Division of Special Education
Department of Education
State House, Room 229
Indianapolis, IN 46204
(317) 232–0570

Department of Human Services
(Vocational Rehabilitation)
P.O. Box 7083
Indianapolis, IN 46207
(317) 232–1147

Division of Developmental
Disabilities
Department of Mental Health
117 East Washington Street
Indianapolis, IN 46204–3647

Iowa

LDA of Iowa
2819 48th Street
Des Moines, IA 50310
(515) 277–4266

Special Education Division
Department of Public
Instruction
Grimes State Office Building
Des Moines, IA 50319
(515) 281–3176

Division of Vocational
Rehabilitation Services
Department of Public Instruction
510 East 12th Street

Des Moines, IA 50319
(515) 281–4348

Governor's Planning Council for
Developmental Disabilities
Department of Human Services
Hoover Building, 5th Floor
Des Moines, IA 50319
(515) 281–3758

Iowa Protection and Advocacy
Services, Inc.
3015 Merle Hay Road, Suite 6
Des Moines, IA 50310
(515) 278–2502

Iowa University Affiliated Facility
Division of Developmental
Disabilities
University Hospital School
University of Iowa
Iowa City, IA 52242
(319) 353–6390

Kansas

Kansas Association for Children
with Learning Disabilities
6536 Maple
Mission, KS 66202
(913) 362–9535

Special Education
Department of Education
120 East 10th Street
Topeka, KS 66612
(913) 296–4945

Special Education Administration
(Ages 3–5)
Department of Education
120 East 10th Street
Topeka, KS 66612
(913) 296–7454

74

Rehabilitation Service
Department of Social and
  Rehabilitation Services
State Office Building
300 SW Oakley,
1st Floor
Topeka, KS 66606
(913) 296–3911

Child and Adolescent Mental
  Health Programs
506 North State Office Building
Topeka, KS 66612
(913) 296–1808

Kansas Planning Council on
  Developmental Disabilities
State Office Building
300 SW Oakley, 1st Floor
Topeka, KS 66606
(913) 296–2608

Kansas Advocacy and Protection
  Services
513 Leavenworth Street,
Suite 2
Manhatten, KS 66502
(913) 776–1541; (800) 432–8276

Kansas University Affiliated
  Faculty
Children's Rehabilitation Unit
Kansas University Medical Center
39th and Rainbow Boulevard
Kansas City, KS 66103
(913) 588–5900

Kansas University Affiliated
  Faculty
348 Haworth Hall
University of Kansas
Lawrence, KS 66045
(913) 864–4950

Kentucky
Association for Children with
  Learning Disabilities (ACLD)
Box 13 B
Battletown, KY 40104
(502) 497–4643

ACLU State Office
2232 Alta Avenue
Louisville, KY 40205
(502) 451–8001

Office of Education for
  Exceptional Children
Department of Education
Capitol Plaza Tower,
8th Floor
Frankfort, KY 40601
(502) 564–4970

Office of Vocational
  Rehabilitation
Department of Education
Capitol Plaza Tower, 9th Floor
Frankfort, KY 40601
(502) 564–4566

Children and Youth Services
  Branch
Department for Mental Health
  and Mental Retardation
  Services
275 East Main Street, 1st Floor
  East
Frankfort, KY 40621
(502) 564–7610

Kentucky Developmental
  Disabilities Planning Council
Bureau of Health Services
275 East Main Street
Frankfort, KY 40621
(502) 564–7842

Office for Public Advocacy
Division for Protection Advocacy
1264 Louisville Road
Frankfort, KY 40601
(502) 564–2967; (800) 373–2988

Interdisciplinary Human
  Development Institute
University Affiliated Facility
University of Kentucky
114 Porter Building
730 South Limestone
Lexington, KY 40506–0205
(606) 257–1714

Louisiana

Association for Children with
  Learning Disabilities (ACLD)
8602 Hollow Bluff Drive
Haughton, LA 71037
(318) 949–2302

Special Education Services
Department of Education
P.O. Box 94064, 9th Floor
Baton Rouge, LA 70864–9064
(504) 342–3633

Division of Vocational
  Rehabilitation
Office of Human Development
1755 Florida Boulevard
P.O. Box 94371
Baton Rouge, LA 70804
(504) 342–2285

Office of Mental Health
Department of Health and
  Human Resources
P.O. Box 4049, 655 North 5th
  Street
Baton Rouge, LA 70821
(504) 342–2548

Maine

LDA of Maine
Bessey Ridge Road
Albion, ME 04901
(207) 437–9245

Division of Special Education
Department of Education and
  Cultural Services
State House, Station 23
Augusta, ME 04333
(207) 289–5953

Bureau of Rehabilitation Services
32 Winthrop Street
Augusta, ME 04330
(207) 289–2266

Department of Mental Health
  and Mental Retardation
411 State Officers Building
Station 40
Augusta, ME 04333
(207) 289–4223

Bureau of Children with Special
  Needs
Department of Mental Health
  and Mental Retardation
411 State Officers Building,
Room 424
Augusta, ME 04333
(207) 289–4250

Developmental Disabilities
  Council
Nash Building, STA 139
Capitol and State Streets
Augusta, ME 04330
(207) 289–4213

University Affiliated Handicapped
  Children's Program

Eastern Maine Medical Center
417 State Street, Box 17
Bangor, ME 04401
(207) 945–7572

Maryland
Association for Children with
  Learning Disabilities
2919 Georgia Avenue
Baltimore, MD 21227
(410) 636–3852

ACLD State Office
320 Maryland National Bank
  Building
Baltimore, MD 21202

Division of Special Education
Department of Education
200 West Baltimore Street
Baltimore, MD 21201
(410) 333–2490

Program Development and
  Assistance Branch (Ages 3–5)
Division of Special Education
200 West Baltimore Street
Baltimore, MD 21201
(410) 333–2495

Division of Vocational
  Rehabilitation
Department of Education
2301 Argonne Drive
Baltimore, MD 21218
(410) 554–3000

Developmental Disabilities
  Administration
Department of Health and
  Mental Hygiene
201 West Preston Street
4th Floor, O'Connor Building

Baltimore, MD 21201
(410) 225–5600

Maryland Developmental
  Disabilities Planning Council
300 West Lexington Street
Baltimore, MD 21201
(410) 333–3688

Massachusetts
Association for Children with
  Learning Disabilities
37 Sleigh Road
Chelmsford, MA 01824
(508) 256–9598

ACLD State Office
P.O. Box 28
West Newton, MA 02165
(617) 891–5009

Division of Special Education
Department of Education
1385 Hancock Street, 3rd Floor
Quincy, MA 02169–5183
(617) 770–7648

Early Childhood Special
  Education (Ages 3–5)
Department of Education
1385 Hancock Street
Quincy, MA 02169
(617) 770–7476

Massachusetts Rehabilitation
  Commission
fort Point Place
27–43 Wormwood Street
Boston, MA 02210
(617) 727–2172

Child-Adolescent Services
Department of Mental Health

24 Farnsworth Street
Boston, MA 02210
(617) 727–5600

Massachusetts Developmental
   Disabilities Planning Council
600 Washington Street,
Room 670
Boston, MA 02111–1704
(617) 727–6374

Client Assistance Program
Massachusetts Office of
   Handicapped Affairs
One Ashburton Place,
Room 303
Boston, MA 02108
(617) 727–7440

Michigan
Association for Children with
   Learning Disabilities (ACLD)
8123 East 9 Mile Road
Big Rapids, MI 49307
(616) 796–8968

Michigan ACLD
P.O. Box 12336
Lansing, MI 48901
(517) 485–8160

Special Education Services
Michigan Department of
   Education
P.O. Box 30008
Lansing, MI 48909
(517) 373–9433

Special Education Services
   (Ages 3–5)
Michigan Department of
   Education
P.O. Box 30008

Lansing, MI 48909
(517) 373–8215

Bureau of Rehabilitation
Department of Education
101 Pine Street, 4th floor
P.O. Box 30010
Lansing, MI 48909
(517) 373–3391

Michigan Developmental
   Disabilities Council
Lewis Cass Building, 6th Floor
Lansing, MI 48926
(517) 373–0341

Michigan Protection and
   Advocacy Service
109 West Michigan, Suite 900
Lansing, MI 48933
(517) 487–1755

University Affiliated Facility
Developmental Disabilities
   Institute
Wayne State University
6001 Cass Avenue
Detroit, MI 48202
(313) 577–2654

Minnesota
Minnesota Association for
   Children with Learning
   Disabilities (ACLD)
541 Southwood Drive
Bloomington, MN 55437
(612) 831–1131

ACLD State Office
1821 University Avenue
Room 494–N
Saint Paul, MN 55104
(612) 646–6136

78

Special Education Section
Department of Education
812 Capitol Square Building
550 Cedar Street
Saint Paul, MN 55101–2233
(612) 296–1793

Division of Vocational
   Rehabilitation
Department of Jobs and Training
390 North Robert Street,
5th Floor
Saint Paul, MN 55101
(612) 296–2962

Division for Persons with
   Developmental Disabilities
444 Lafayette Road
Saint Paul, MN 55155
(612) 297–0307

Governor's Planning Council on
   Developmental Disabilities
658 Cedar Street,
Room 300
Saint Paul, MN 55155
(612) 296–4018

University Affiliated Program on
   Developmental Disabilities
University of Minnesota
6 Patte Hall
Minneapolis, MN 55455
(612) 624–4848

Mississippi
LDA of Mississippi
Rt. 2, Box 110
Minter City, MS 38944
(601) 453–3600

LDA State Office
P.O. Box 9386

Jackson, MS 39206
(601) 982–2812

Bureau of Special Services
Department of Education
P.O. Box 771
Jackson, MS 39205–0771
(601) 359–3490

Department of Vocational
   Services
P.O. Box 1698
Jackson, MS 39205
(601) 354–6825

Mississippi Developmental
   Disability Planning Council
1101 Robert E. Lee Building
Jackson, MS 39201
(601) 359–1290

Mississippi Protection and
   Advocacy System for
   Developmentally Disabled, Inc.
4793 East McWille Drive
Jackson, MS 39206
(601) 981–8207

Mississippi University Affiliated
   Program
University of Southern Mississippi
Southern Station, Box 5163
Hattiesburg, MS 34906–5163
(601) 266–5163

Missouri
LDA of Missouri
6153 Holmes
Kansas City, MO 64110
(816) 363–5844

LDA State Office
P.O. Box 3302

1918 East Meadowmere, #10
Springfield, MO 65808
(417) 864–5110

Division of Special Education
Department of Elementary and
  Secondary Education
P.O. Box 480
Jefferson City, MO 65102
(314) 751–2965

Division of Special Education
Department of Elementary and
  Secondary Education
  (Ages 3–5)
P.O. Box 480
Jefferson City, MO 65102
(314) 751–0185

Division of Vocational
  Rehabilitation
Department of Education
2401 East McCarty Street
Jefferson City, MO 65101
(314) 751–3251

Children and Youth Services
Department of Mental Health
P.O. Box 687
Jefferson City, MO 65102
(314) 751–9482

Missouri Planning Council for
  Developmental Disabilities
P.O. Box 687
Jefferson City, MO 65102
(314) 751–4054

Missouri Protection and
  Advocacy Services
925 South Country Club Drive,
  Unit B–1
Jefferson City, MO 65109

(314) 893–3333;
(800) 392–8667

University Affiliated Program for
  Developmental Disabilities
University of Missouri at Kansas
  City
Institute for Human
  Development
2220 Holmes Street
Kansas City, MO 64108
(816) 276–1770

Montana
Montana Association for
  Children with Learning
  Disabilities (ACLD)
2535 35th Street, SE
Harve, MT 59501
(406) 265–5633

Special Education Division
Office of Public Instruction
State Capitol, Room 106
Helena, MT 59602
(406) 444–4429

Department of Education
  Services (Ages 3–5)
Office of Public Instruction
State Capitol
Helena, MT 59602
(406) 444–4428

Rehabilitation Services Division
Department of Social and
  Rehabilitation Services
P.O. Box 4210
Helena, MT 59601
(406) 444–2590

Division of Developmental
  Disabilities

Department of Social and
  Rehabilitation Services
P.O. Box 4210
111 Sanders, Room 202
Helena, MT 59604
(406) 444–2995

Montana Center for Handicapped
  Children
Eastern Montana College
1500 North 30th Street
Billings, MT 59101–0298
(406) 657–2312

Nebraska

Association for Children with
  Learning Disabilities (ACLD)
5835 Corby
Omaha, NE 68104

Special Education Branch
Department of Education
P.O. Box 94987
301 Centennial Mall South
Lincoln, NE 68509
(402) 471–2471

Jan Thelen, Coordinator
Division of Rehabilitation
  Services
Department of Education
P.O. Box 94987
301 Centennial Mall,
6th Floor
Lincoln, NE 68509
(402) 471–2961

Department of
  Health/Developmental
  Disabilities
P.O. Box 95007
Lincoln, NE 68509
(402) 471–2330

Nebraska Advocacy Services
522 Lincoln Central Building
215 Centennial Mall South
Lincoln, NE 68508
(402) 474–3183

Nevada

Special Education
Department of Education
State Capitol Complex
400 West King Street
Carson City, NV 89710
(702) 687–3140

Special Education Branch
  (Ages 3–5)
Department of Education
State Capitol Complex
400 West King Street
Carson City, NV 89710
(702) 885–3140

Rehabilitation Division
Department of Human Resources
State Capitol Complex
505 East King Street
Carson City, NV 89710
(702) 687–4452

Developmental Disabilities
  Council
State Capitol Complex
505 East King Street,
Room 502
Carson City, NV 89710–0001
(702) 687–4452

Office of Protection and
  Advocacy
2105 Capurro Way, Suite B
Sparks, NV 89431
(702) 789–0233;
(800) 992–5715

New Hampshire

New Hampshire Association for
  Children with Learning
  Disabilities (ACLD)
20 Wedgewood Drive
Concord, NH 03307
(603) 224–5872

Special Education Bureau
Department of Education
101 Pleasant Street
Concord, NH 03301–3860
(603) 271–3741

Division of Mental Health and
  Developmental Services
Department of Health and
  Welfare
State Office Park South
105 Pleasant Street
Concord, NH 03301
(603) 271–5013

Disabilities Rights Center
P.O. Box 19
Concord, NH 03302–0019
(603) 228–0432

Parent Information Center
155 Manchester Street
P.O. Box 1422
Concord, NH 03302–1422
(603) 224–6299

New Jersey

Association for Children with
  Learning Disabilities (ACLD)
305 North Lancaster Avenue
Margate, NJ 08402
 (609) 823–5608

ACLD State Office
640 Ocean Avenue

West End, NJ 07740
(201) 229–1919

Division of Special Education
Department of Education
225 West State Street, CN 500
Trenton, NJ 08615
(609) 633–6833

Division of Developmental
  Disabilities
Department of Labor and
  Industry
1005 Labor and Industry
  Building, CN 398
John Fitch Plaza
Trenton, NJ 08625

Division of Developmental
  Disabilities
Department of Human Services
2–98 East State Street, CN 726
Trenton, NJ 08625
(609) 292–7260

Bureau of Children's Services
Division of Mental Health and
  Hospitals
Capital Center, CN 727
Trenton, NJ 08625
(609) 777–0702

New Jersey Developmental
  Disability Council
108–110 North Broadway Street,
  CN 700
Trenton, NJ 08625
(609) 292–3745

Department of Public Advocate
Office of Advocacy for the
  Developmentally Disabled
Hughes Justice Complex, CN 850

Trenton, NJ 08625
(609) 292–1750;
(800) 792–8600

University Affiliated Facility
University of Medicine and
  Dentistry of New Jersey
Robert W. Johnson Medical
  School
675 Hoes Lane
Piscataway, NJ 08854–5635
(201) 463–4447

New Mexico
New Mexico ACLD
824 Vassar Drive
Albuquerque, NM 87106
(505) 255–9324

Special Education Unit
Department of Education
Education Building
300 Don Gasper Avenue
Santa Fe, NM 87501–2786
(505) 827–6541

Division of Vocational
  Rehabilitation
Department of Education
604 West San Mateo
Santa Fe, NM 87503
(505) 827–3511

Community Programs
Department of Health and the
  Environment
1190 Street Francis Drive
Santa Fe, NM 87503
(505) 827–2573

New Mexico Developmental
  Disabilities Planning Council
2025 Pacheco Street,

Suite 200–B
Santa Fe, NM 87505
(505) 827–2707

New York
New York ALD
8 Weiser Street
Glenmont, NY 12077
(518) 783–1644

ALD State Office
90 South Swan Street
Albany, NY 12210
(518) 436–4633

Office of Education of Children
  with Handicapping Conditions
Department of Education
1073 Education Building Annex
Albany, NY 12234–0001
(518) 474–5548

Office of Education of Children
  with Handicapping Conditions
  (Ages 3–5)
Department of Education
1073 Education Building Annex
Albany, NY 12234–0001
(518) 474–8917

Office of Vocational
  Rehabilitation
Department of Education
One Commerce Plaza,
16th Floor
Albany, NY 12234
(518) 474–2714

Office of Mental Retardation and
  Developmental Disabilities
44 Holland Avenue
Albany, NY 12229
(518) 473–1997

83

Bureau of Children and Families
Office of Mental Health
44 Holland Avenue
Albany, NY 12229
(518) 474–6902

New York State Developmental
  Disabilities Planning Council
155 Washington Avenue,
2nd Floor
Albany, NY 12210
(518) 432–8233

University Affiliated Facility
Rose F. Kennedy Center
Albert Einstein College of
  Medicine
Yeshiva University
1410 Pelham Parkway
South Bronx, NY 10461
(212) 430–2325

University Affiliated Program for
  Developmental Disabilities
University of Rochester Medical
  Center
601 Elmwood Avenue
Rochester, NY 14642
(716) 275–2986

North Carolina
LDA of North Carolina
510 Colony Woods Drive
Chapel Hill, NC 27514
(919) 966–4041

LDA State Office
Box 3542
Chapel Hill, NC 27514
(919) 967–9537

Division for Exceptional Children
Department of Public Instruction

Education Building,
Room 442
116 West Edenton
Raleigh, NC 27603
(919) 733–3921

Division of Vocational
  Rehabilitation
Department of Human Resources
620 North West Street
Raleigh, NC 27611
(919) 733–3364

North Carolina Council on
  Developmental Disabilities
1508 Western Boulevard
Raleigh, NC 27606
(919) 733–6566

Governor's Advocacy Council for
  Persons with Disabilities
1318 Dale Street, Suite 100
Raleigh, NC 27605
(919) 733–9250

North Dakota
North Dakota Association for
  Children and Adults with
  Learning Disabilities (ACLD)
P.O. Box 814
Fargo, ND 58107
(701) 293–7914

Special Education Division
Department of Public Instruction
600 East Boulevard
Bismarck, ND 58505
(701) 224–2277

Department of Vocational
  Rehabilitation
State Board of Social Services
State Capitol Building

Bismarck, ND 58505
(701) 224–2907

Developmental Disabilities
  Division
Department of Human Services
State Capitol Building
600 East Boulevard
Bismarck, ND 58505
(701) 224–2907

North Dakota Developmental
  Disabilities Council
Department of Human Services
State Capitol Building
Bismarck, ND 58505
(701) 224–2970

Ohio

Ohio Association for Children
  and Adults with Learning
  Disabilities (ACLD)
2874 Castlewood Road
Columbus, OH 43209
(614) 231–3321

ACLD State Office
1480 Pearl Road, #5
Brunswick, OH 44212
(216) 273–7388

Division of Special Education
Department of Education
933 High Street
Worthington, OH 43085–4017
(614) 466–2650

Early Childhood Section (Ages
  3–5)
Department of Education
65 South Front Street, Room 202
Columbus, OH 43266
(614) 466–0224

Rehabilitation Services
  Commission
400 East Campus View Boulevard
Columbus, OH 43235
(614) 438–1210

Department of Mental
  Retardation and Development
  Disabilities
State Office Tower
30 East Broad Street,
Room 1280
Columbus, OH 43224
(614) 466–5214

Oklahoma

Oklahoma Association for
  Children and Adults with
  Learning Disabilities (ACLD)
1701 Leawood Drive
Edmond, OK 73034
(405) 341–2980, ext. 2236

ACLD State Office
3701 NW 62nd Street
Oklahoma City, OK 73112
(405) 943–9434

Special Education Division
Department of Education
Oliver Hodge Memorial Building,
Room 215
Oklahoma City, OK 73105–4599
(405) 521–3351

Rehabilitation Services Division
2409 North Kelley
Oklahoma City, OK 73125
(405) 424–6006, ext. 2840

Developmental Disability Services
Department of Human Services
P.O. Box 25352

Oklahoma City, OK 73125
(405) 521–3571

Oklahoma Developmental
  Disability Planning Council
Box 25352
Oklahoma City, OK 73125
(405) 521–4984

Protection and Advocacy Agency
Osage Building, Room 133
9726 East 42nd Street
Tulsa, OK 74146
(918) 664–5883

Oregon
Special Education and Student
  Services Division
Department of Education
700 Pringle Parkway, SE
Salem, OR 97310
(503) 378–3591

Division of Special Education
  (Ages 3–5)
Department of Education
700 Pringle Parkway, SE
Salem, OR 97301
(503) 373–1484

Vocational Rehabilitation
  Division
Department of Human Resources
2045 Silverton Road, NE
Salem, OR 97310
(503) 378–3830

Program for Mental Retardation
  and Developmental Disabilities
Department of Human Resources
2575 Bittern Street, NW
Salem, OR 97310
(503) 378–2429

Oregon Developmental
  Disabilities Planning Council
540 24th Place, NE
Salem, OR 97301
(503) 373–7555

Pennsylvania
Pennsylvania ACLD
2551 West 8th Street
Erie, PA 16505
(814) 838–1966, ext. 303

Bureau of Special Education
Department of Education
333 Market Street
Harrisburg, PA 17126–0333
(717) 783–6913

Bureau of Vocational
  Rehabilitation
Department of Labor and
  Industry
Labor and Industry Building,
  Room 1300
7th and Forster Streets
Harrisburg, PA 17120
(717) 787–5244

Developmental Disabilities
  Planning Council
forum Building, Room 569
Commonwealth Avenue
Harrisburg, PA 17120
(717) 787–6057

Protection and Advocacy, Inc.
116 Pine Street
Harrisburg, PA 17101
(717) 323–8110; (800) 692–7443

Developmental Disabilities
  Program
Temple University

9th Floor, Ritter Annex
13th Street and Cecil Moore
  Avenue
Philadelphia, PA 19122
(215) 787–1356

Rhode Island
Rhode Island Association for
  Children and Adults with
  Learning Disabilities (ACLD)
103 Harris Avenue
Johnston, RI 02919
(401) 461–0820, ext. 539

Special Education Program
Department of Education
Roger Williams Building,
Room 209
22 Hayes Street
Providence, RI 02908
(401) 277–3505

Vocational Rehabilitation
Department of Human Services
40 Fountain Street
Providence, RI 02903
(401) 421–7005

Rhode Island Developmental
  Disabilities Council
600 New London Avenue
Cranston, RI 02920
(401) 464–3191

Rhode Island Protection and
  Advocacy System, Inc.
55 Bradford Street,
2nd Floor
Providence, RI 02903
(401) 831–3150

Child Development Center
Rhode Island Hospital

593 Eddy Street
Providence, RI 02920
(401) 277–5681

South Carolina
South Carolina Association for
  Children and
Adults with Learning Disabilities
  (ACLD)
1792 Sharonwood Lane
Rock Hill, SC 29730
(803) 366–4141 (W)

Office of Programs for the
  Handicapped
Department of Education
Santee Building, A–24
100 Executive Center Drive
Columbia, SC 29201
(803) 737–7810

Vocational Rehabilitation
  Department
1410 Boston Ave
P.O. Box 15
West Columbia, SC 29171
(803) 734–4300

South Carolina Developmental
  Disability Planning Council
1205 Pendleton Street,
Room 372
Columbia, SC 29201
(803) 734–0465

South Carolina Protection and
  Advocacy System for the
  Handicapped, Inc.
3710 Landmark Drive, Suite 208
Columbia, SC 29204

University Affiliated Facility of
  South Carolina

Center for Developmental
  Disabilities
Benson Building,
Pickens Street
University of South Carolina
Columbia, SC 29208
(803) 777–4839

South Dakota
LDA of South Dakota
4022 Helen Court
Rapid City, SD 57701
(605) 343–4320

Section for Special Education
Department of Education
Kneip Office Building
700 North Illinois Street
Pierre, SD 57501
(605) 773–3315

Section for Special Education
  (Ages 3-5)
Department of Education and
  Cultural Affairs
700 North Governors Drive
Pierre, SD 57501
(605) 773–4329

Division of Rehabilitation
  Services
700 North Governors Drive
Pierre, SD 57501
(605) 773–3195

Developmental Disabilities and
  Mental Health
700 North Illinois Street
Pierre, SD 57501
(605) 733–3438

University of South Dakota
  Affiliated Facility

Center for Developmental
  Disabilities
U.S.D. School of Medicine
Vermillion, SD 57069
(605) 677–5311

Tennessee
Special Education Programs
Department of Education
132 Cordell Hull Building
Nashville, TN 37219

Division of Vocational
  Rehabilitation
Department of Human Services
400 Deaderick Street, 15th Floor
Nashville, TN 37219
(615) 741–2521

Office of Children and Adolescent
  Services
Doctors Building
706 Church Street
Nashville, TN 37219
(615) 741–3708

Center for Developmental
  Disabilities
University of Tennessee, Memphis
711 Jefferson Avenue
Memphis, TN 38105
(901) 528–6511

Texas
Texas Association for Children
  and Adults with Learning
  Disabilities (ACLD)
2909 Wildflower
Bryan, TX 77802
(409) 776–2807

ACLD State Office
1011 West 31st Street

88

Austin, TX 78705
(512) 458–8234

Special Education Programs
Texas Education Agency
Wm. B. Travis Building,
Room 5–120
1701 North Congress Avenue
Austin, TX 78701–2486
(512) 463–9414

Texas Rehabilitation Commission
4900 North Lamar
Austin, TX 78751
(512) 483–4001

Children and Youth Mental
  Health Services
Department of Mental Health
  and Mental Retardation
Box 12668, Capitol Station
Austin, TX 78711
(512) 465–4657

Texas Planning Council for
  Developmental Disabilities
4900 North Lamar Boulevard
Austin, TX 78751–2316
(512) 483–4080

Utah
LDA of Utah
2030 East 9100 Street
Sandy, UT 84093
(801) 943–4425

LDA State Office
P.O. Box 112
Salt Lake City, UT 84110
(801) 364–0126

Special Education Section
State Office of Education

250 East 500 South
Salt Lake City, UT 84111–3204
(801) 538–7706

Special Education Section
  (Ages 3–5)
State Office of Education
250 East 500 South
Salt Lake City, UT 84111
(801) 538–7700

Office of Rehabilitation
State Office of Education
250 East 500 South
Salt Lake City, UT 84111
(801) 538–7530

Vermont
Division of Special Education
Department of Education
120 State Street
Montpelier, VT 05602–3403
(802) 828–3141

Vocational Rehabilitation Division
Department of Social and
  Rehabilitation Services
103 South Main Street
Waterbury, VT 05676
(802) 241–2189

Virginia
LDA of Virginia
P.O. Box 717
Woodstock, VA 22664
(703) 459–8804

Special and Compensatory
  Education
Department of Education
P.O. Box 6Q
Richmond, VA 23216–2060
(804) 225–2402

Division of Special Education
  Programs (Ages 3–5)
Department of Education
P.O. Box 6Q
Richmond, VA 23216–2060
(804) 225–2873

Department of Rehabilitation
  Services
State Board of Vocational
  Rehabilitation
P.O. Box 11045
Richmond, VA 23230

Developmental Disability
  Planning Council
Monroe Building,
17th Floor
101 North 14th Street
Richmond, VA 23219
(804) 225–2042

Department for Rights of the
  Disabled
James Monroe Building,
17th Floor
101 North 14th Street
Richmond, VA 23219
(804) 225–2042

Virginia Institute for
  Developmental Disabilities
Virginia Commonwealth
  University
301 West Franklin Street,
Box 3020
Richmond, VA 23284–3020
(804) 224–3876

Washington
LDA of Washington
18921 27th Drive, SE
Bothell, WA 98012

(206) 481–8918
LDA State Office
17530 NW Union Hill,
Suite 100
Redmond, WA 98052
(206) 882–0792

Special Education Section
Superintendent of Public
  Instruction
FG–11 Old Capitol Building
Olympia, WA 98504–0001
(206) 753–6733

Superintendent of Public
  Instruction (Ages 3–5)
FG–11 Old Capitol Building
Olympia, WA 98504
(206) 753–0317

Division of Vocational
  Rehabilitation
Department of Social and Health
  Services
MS: OB–21C
Olympia, WA 98504
(206) 753–2544

Division of Developmental
  Disabilities
Department of Social and Health
  Services
P.O. Box 1788, OB–42C
Olympia, WA 98504
(206) 753–3900

West Virginia
West Virginia Association for
  Children and Adults with
  Learning Disabilities (ACLD)
Rt. 3, Box 70
Mineral Wells, WV 26150
(304) 489–9621

Office of Special Education
Department of Education
B–304, Building 6
Capitol Complex
Charleston, WV 25305
(304) 348–2696

Division of Rehabilitation
  Services
State Board of Rehabilitation
State Capitol
Charleston, WV 25305
(304) 766–4601

Office of Behavioral Health
Department of Health and
  Human Resources
1800 Washington Street, East
Charleston, WV 25305
(304) 348–0627

Developmental Disability
  Planning Council
1601 Kanawha Boulevard,
  West
Charleston, WV 25312
(304) 348–0416

Wisconsin
Wisconsin Association for
  Children and Adults with
  Learning Disabilities (ACLD)
2622 Oak Crest Drive
Neenah, WI 54956
(414) 722–4977

Obsessive Compulsive
  Information Center
University of Wisconsin
Department of Psychiatry
600 Highland Avenue
Madison, WI 53792

Division of Handicapped Children
  and Pupil Services
Department of Public Instruction
125 South Webster Street
P.O. Box 7841
Madison, WI 53707–7841
(608) 266–1649

Early Childhood Handicapped
  Programs (Ages 3–5)
Department of Public Instruction
P.O. Box 7841
Madison, WI 53707
(608) 266–6981

Division of Vocational
  Rehabilitation
Department of Health and Social
  Services
1 West Wilson Street, Room 830
Madison WI 53702
(608) 266–2168

Developmental Disabilities Office
Department of Health and
  Human Services
P.O. Box 7851
Madison, WI 53707
(608) 266–9329

Wisconsin Council on
  Developmental Disabilities
722 Williamson Street,
2nd Floor
Madison, WI 53707
(608) 266–7826

Wyoming
Special Programs Unit
Department of Education
Hathaway Building, 2nd Floor
Cheyenne, WY 82002–0050
(307) 777–7414

Division of Vocational
  Rehabilitation
Department of Employment
1100 Herschler Building
Cheyenne, WY 82002
(307) 777–7385

Division of Community Programs
356 Hathaway Building
Cheyenne, WY 82002
(307) 777–7115

Wyoming Protection and
  Advocacy System, Inc.
2424 Pioneer Avenue, No. 101
Cheyenne, WY 82001
(307) 638–7668

Index

Italicized page numbers indicate illustrations.

Sporadic Tourette Syndrome, 18

Stress, 17, 22, 23, 28

Suicide, 33

Supports groups, 3437, *35, 36*

Swearing. *See* Coprolalia

Tardive dyskinesia, 24

Tics, 12, 13, 17, 18, 21, 22, 25, 34, 35, 37, 38, 48, 54, 57
  complex, 811, *10,* 16
  motor tics, 7, 8, *10,* 15, 16, 20, 21, 24, 29, 30, 45, 46, 56, 57
  simple, 8, *9,* 16
  suppression of, 11, 13, 46, 54, 55
  vocal tics, 711, 1314, 15, 16, 20, 24, 29, 30, 32, 33, 38, 45, 46, 56, 57, 59

Tidmore, Kurt, 59

Toronto, Canada, 53

Tourette, Georges Gilles de la, 15

Tourette and Tic Laboratory and Clinic of the Mount Sinai School of Medicine, 49

Tourette Syndrome Association, 52
  Scientific Advisory Board, 12

Tricyclic antidepressants, 26

29th Street (film), 56

United States, 12

Vocal tics, 711, 1314, 15, 16, 20, 24, 29, 30, 32, 33, 38, 45, 46, 56, 57, 59

Weinberger, Daniel, 17

Young, Ann, 1213

About the Author

Popular author Elaine Landau worked as a newspaper reporter, an editor, and a youth services librarian before becoming a full-time writer. She has written more than ninety nonfiction books for young people, including Alzheimer's Disease and Stalking. Ms. Landau, who has a bachelor's degree in English and journalism from New York University and a master's degree in library and information science from Pratt Institute, lives in Florida with her husband and son.